Type 2 Diabetes Cookbook For Beginners

1800 Days Of Easy And Tasty Recipes For Type 2 Diabetes. Included 45-Day Meal Plan

By Morghy Books

Table Of Contents

Chapter 1: Understanding Type 2 Diabetes

The Basics of Type 2 Diabetes

Embarking on a journey to understand this chronic condition involves unraveling the complexities of how the body manages and utilizes glucose. Normally, glucose serves as a vital energy source, particularly for the brain and muscles. The pancreas plays a crucial role in this process, producing insulin, a hormone that enables glucose to enter cells.

In individuals with this condition, the cells become resistant to insulin, leading to elevated blood glucose levels or hyperglycemia. This imbalance is a precursor to various health complications, including heart disease, kidney damage, and nerve disorders.

Unlike Type 1 Diabetes, which typically has a congenital onset, this variant often develops gradually and is influenced by lifestyle factors. Its insidious nature means it can progress unnoticed, emphasizing the importance of awareness and early detection.

Risk factors intertwine genetics and lifestyle. Family history sets a predisposition, but diet, activity levels, and weight significantly impact its development. Excess weight, particularly abdominal fat, is a notable risk enhancer.

Diagnosis usually follows routine blood tests, with the A1C test being a common method. This test measures average blood sugar levels over months, with an A1C level of 6.5% or higher on two separate tests indicating diabetes. Fasting blood sugar tests and glucose tolerance tests are also employed.

Symptoms may be subtle initially, including increased thirst, frequent urination, hunger, and fatigue. In some cases, the condition is only detected after complications have arisen, underscoring the importance of proactive health monitoring.

Management requires a multifaceted approach. Dietary adjustments, increased physical activity, and weight management are foundational strategies. For some, medications or insulin therapy may be necessary to maintain balanced glucose levels.

Interestingly, this condition is no longer confined to mature adults. Shifts in lifestyle and increasing obesity rates have seen its prevalence rise in younger populations, highlighting the need for early education on healthy living.

Navigating the sea of information surrounding this condition demands discernment. It's essential to separate facts from myths and base understanding on scientific evidence and clinical expertise.

How Diet Affects Diabetes

Understanding this interplay is crucial for anyone navigating the waters of diabetes management.

Carbohydrates, often the center of many dietary discussions, play a pivotal role. Found in foods like fruits, vegetables, grains, and dairy products, carbohydrates break down into glucose, entering the bloodstream and affecting blood sugar levels. For someone with diabetes, it's not just about avoiding sugar; it's about understanding the types of carbohydrates consumed. Complex carbohydrates, such as whole grains and fibrous vegetables, are metabolized slower than simple sugars, leading to a more gradual rise in blood sugar.

But the story doesn't end with carbohydrates. Protein and fats also play significant roles. Protein is essential for muscle and tissue repair and doesn't directly raise blood sugar levels, but it should be consumed in moderation. Fats, especially healthy fats like those found in avocados and nuts, are crucial for overall health but should be balanced to avoid weight gain, a significant risk factor in diabetes management.

Meal timing and portion control are equally vital. Regular, balanced meals help maintain steady blood sugar levels, preventing the peaks and valleys that can occur with irregular eating patterns. Portion sizes directly affect glucose levels and managing them is key to preventing overconsumption of carbohydrates.

The glycemic index (GI) of foods is another important consideration. This measure reflects how quickly foods raise blood sugar levels. Foods with a low GI, such as most fruits and non-starchy vegetables, have a lesser impact on blood sugar spikes, whereas high GI foods, like white bread and sugary snacks, cause rapid increases.

Hydration also plays a crucial role. Water is the best choice, as it doesn't raise blood sugar levels. Sugary drinks, including sodas and fruit juices, can lead to significant sugar spikes and should be consumed sparingly, if at all.

Understanding nutritional labels is an essential skill in this dietary dance. It allows for informed decisions about what foods to include and how much to consume, enabling a person to manage their condition effectively.

Dietary management doesn't mean living in deprivation. It's about making informed, mindful choices. Replacing refined carbohydrates with whole grains, incorporating more fruits and vegetables, choosing lean proteins, and opting for healthy fats are all part of a balanced approach.

Moreover, individualized dietary planning is crucial. What works for one person may not work for another. Factors like age, activity level, weight, and medication must be considered when developing a meal plan. Consulting with a dietitian or healthcare provider can provide tailored advice that aligns with personal health goals and dietary preferences.

Myths and Facts

Navigating the world of diabetes is often clouded by a myriad of myths and misconceptions. These can range from outdated beliefs to oversimplified notions about the disease. Dispelling these myths is essential for a clear and accurate understanding of diabetes management.

Myth 1: Eating Too Much Sugar Causes Diabetes

One of the most prevalent misconceptions is that consuming excessive sugar directly leads to diabetes. While a diet high in calories, sugar, and unhealthy fats can contribute to obesity – a significant risk factor for Type 2 Diabetes – sugar alone is not the sole culprit. The development of this condition is a complex interplay of genetic, environmental, and lifestyle factors.

Myth 2: People with Diabetes Can't Eat Carbohydrates

Another common fallacy is the belief that individuals with diabetes must completely avoid carbohydrates. Carbohydrates are a vital part of a balanced diet and provide necessary energy. The key is to choose complex carbohydrates, like whole grains, and to be mindful of portion sizes, ensuring a balanced intake that doesn't cause blood sugar levels to spike.

Myth 3: Diabetes Is Not a Serious Condition

Often, people underestimate the severity of diabetes, considering it less serious than other chronic conditions. This underestimation can lead to a lack of urgency in managing the disease. In reality, when not managed properly, diabetes can lead to severe complications such as heart disease, kidney failure, and nerve damage.

Myth 4: Insulin Injections Mean You Have Failed

For some, the need to start insulin therapy is seen as a personal failure in managing diabetes. This belief can be damaging and misleading. Insulin therapy is simply another method of treatment and, for some, an essential step in effectively managing their diabetes. It's not a failure but an adjustment in treatment strategy.

Myth 5: Diabetic Diets Are Highly Restrictive

The idea that a diabetes-friendly diet is extremely restrictive is another myth. While it's true that careful consideration is needed in meal planning, a diabetic diet can be diverse and full of flavor. It involves choosing healthier options, balancing meal components, and understanding how different foods affect blood sugar levels.

Myth 6: If You Are Overweight, You Will Inevitably Develop Diabetes

While obesity is a significant risk factor for Type 2 Diabetes, it is not a definitive predictor. Many individuals who are overweight never develop diabetes, and many with diabetes are of normal weight. It's a complex condition influenced by multiple factors beyond body weight.

Myth 7: Diabetes Only Affects People of a Certain Age

Initially thought to be a condition only affecting older adults, current trends show that Type 2 Diabetes can occur at any age, largely influenced by lifestyle choices, obesity, and genetics. This shift underscores the importance of healthy living at all stages of life.

Myth 8: Natural Sweeteners Are Always Better

Replacing refined sugar with natural sweeteners is often seen as a safer option for diabetes. While natural sweeteners like honey or maple syrup have nutritional benefits, they still impact blood sugar levels and should be used in moderation.

Understanding the facts behind these myths is crucial for effective diabetes management.

Chapter 2: The Role of Nutrition in Managing Diabetes

Essential Nutrients for Diabetics

In the realm of managing Type 2 Diabetes, nutrition holds a place of unparalleled importance. It's not merely about sustenance but about harnessing the power of food as a tool to balance and regulate blood sugar levels. The right nutrients can act as allies in this ongoing endeavor, each playing a unique role in the broader strategy of diabetes management.

At the heart of this nutritional approach is understanding that not all foods are created equal in their impact on blood sugar levels and overall health. Carbohydrates, often vilified in the world of diabetes management, are not inherently adverse. However, their type and quantity play a pivotal role. Complex carbohydrates, found in whole grains, legumes, and fibrous vegetables, are metabolized more slowly, providing a steady source of energy without causing abrupt spikes in blood sugar. In contrast, simple carbohydrates, prevalent in sugary snacks and refined grains, can lead to rapid increases in glucose levels.

Diving deeper into the world of carbohydrates, fiber emerges as a star player. This indigestible part of plant foods aids in slowing the absorption of sugar, thus assisting in maintaining steadier blood glucose levels. High-fiber foods like beans, whole grains, and a variety of fruits and vegetables not only support blood sugar management but also contribute to heart health—a critical consideration, given the increased risk of cardiovascular issues in individuals with diabetes.

Proteins, the building blocks of life, are integral to a balanced diabetic diet. Lean proteins, such as poultry, fish, tofu, and legumes, provide essential nutrients without the added burden of excessive saturated fats. Importantly, proteins have minimal impact on blood glucose levels, making them a key component in meal planning. They contribute to a sense of fullness, reducing the likelihood of overeating and aiding in weight management, a crucial aspect of diabetes care.

Fats, often misunderstood, are necessary for overall health but require careful selection and moderation. Monounsaturated and polyunsaturated fats, found in foods like avocados, nuts, seeds, and olive oil, can promote heart health and provide sustained energy. These healthier fats can also aid in the absorption of vitamins and provide a sense of satiety. However, it's vital to limit the intake of saturated and trans fats, commonly found in fried foods, processed snacks, and baked goods, as they can exacerbate heart disease risk.

Micronutrients, though required in smaller amounts, are vital cogs in the machinery of health. Vitamins and minerals like magnesium, potassium, vitamin D, and B vitamins play various roles, from supporting nerve function to enhancing energy metabolism. A diet rich in a variety of vegetables, fruits, whole grains, and lean proteins can provide these essential nutrients.

Hydration also plays a critical role in diabetes management. Water, the elixir of life, helps regulate body temperature, supports kidney function, and aids in the removal of waste products. For individuals with diabetes, staying hydrated is key in helping manage blood sugar levels and reducing the risk of complications. Unlike sugary beverages, which can cause blood sugar levels to spike, water provides hydration without the added risk.

Meal planning and portion control are foundational in managing diabetes with nutrition. It's not just about choosing the right foods but also about consuming them in the right amounts and combinations. Balancing meals with appropriate portions of carbohydrates, proteins, and fats can help maintain stable blood sugar levels and support overall health. This approach requires mindfulness and sometimes a shift in long-standing eating habits, but the rewards in health and well-being are substantial.

For individuals with diabetes, understanding the glycemic index and glycemic load of foods can be particularly beneficial. These measures indicate how foods affect blood sugar levels. Foods with a low glycemic index, like lentils, quinoa, and non-starchy vegetables, have a more moderate impact on blood sugar, whereas high-glycemic foods, such as white bread and short-grain rice, can cause rapid spikes. Incorporating low-glycemic foods into meals can lead to more stable blood sugar levels throughout the day.

Equally important in diabetes management is understanding the impact of meals on blood sugar levels. Keeping a food diary can be an effective tool in identifying how different foods and meals affect individual blood sugar readings. This personalized approach to nutrition allows for more tailored and effective meal planning.

Reading Food Labels

Food labels are like maps, providing valuable information about what's inside the packaging. They offer insights into the nutritional content of food items, helping individuals with diabetes to make choices that align with their dietary needs. Understanding these labels is not just about reading numbers; it's about comprehending what those numbers mean in the context of a diabetes-friendly diet. At the forefront of a food label is the serving size. This often-overlooked detail is the key to interpreting the rest of the information correctly. Serving sizes are standardized to make it easier to compare similar foods, but they may not always match the portion size one might typically eat. It's crucial to adjust the rest of the nutritional information based on the actual amount consumed.

Calories, listed next on most labels, are a measure of the amount of energy provided by the food. For individuals managing diabetes and perhaps also watching their weight, understanding calorie intake is important. However, the quality of the calories matters as much as the quantity. Calories from nutrient-rich foods will have a different impact on health than those from foods high in sugar and unhealthy fats.

Carbohydrates, the nutrient with the most direct impact on blood sugar levels, are broken down into three categories on labels: total carbohydrates, dietary fiber, and sugars. For diabetes management, focusing on the total carbohydrate count is more crucial than just the sugar content. This total includes all types of carbohydrates in the food, providing a more accurate picture of its potential impact on blood sugar. Dietary fiber, a type of carbohydrate not digested by the body, can help regulate blood sugar levels and should be considered in the context of total carbohydrate intake.

Proteins and fats are also listed on the label. While they have less direct impact on blood sugar than carbohydrates, they are important for overall nutrition and satiety. Healthy fats, particularly unsaturated fats, should be chosen over saturated and trans fats to support heart health.

Another section of the label worth noting is the percent daily value (%DV). This number indicates how much a nutrient in a serving of food contributes to a daily diet. For individuals with diabetes, %DV can help gauge if a food is high or low in nutrients like dietary fiber, vitamins, minerals, or unhealthy fats.

In addition to these basic components, food labels also list ingredients. Ingredients are listed in order of quantity, from highest to lowest. This list is crucial for identifying added sugars, unhealthy fats, and other ingredients that might be best avoided. Terms like 'sucrose', 'high-fructose corn syrup', 'hydrogenated oils', and 'shortening' can flag foods potentially detrimental to diabetes management.

Understanding food labels also means being aware of marketing tactics. Terms like 'low-fat', 'reduced sugar', or 'multigrain' can be misleading. For example, 'low-fat' foods may still be high in calories and carbohydrates, and 'multigrain' does not necessarily mean whole grain.

For someone with diabetes, mastering the art of label reading is empowering. It turns grocery shopping into an informed activity, aligning choices with the goals of managing blood sugar levels, maintaining a healthy weight, and overall well-being.

Balancing Carbs, Proteins, and Fats

The art of managing diabetes lies significantly in the balancing act of macronutrients - carbohydrates, proteins, and fats. This equilibrium is not just a dietary goal but a crucial factor in maintaining stable blood sugar levels and overall health. The interplay of these nutrients influences how the body processes food, uses energy, and controls blood glucose levels.

Carbohydrates: The Energy Regulators

Carbohydrates are often the primary focus in diabetes management due to their direct impact on blood sugar levels. The key is not to eliminate them but to choose them wisely and balance their intake. Carbohydrates are found in foods like fruits, vegetables, grains, and dairy products. The objective is to opt for complex carbohydrates, such as whole grains, legumes, and fibrous vegetables, over simple carbohydrates found in sugary foods and refined grains.

The amount of carbohydrates consumed at each meal will vary depending on individual factors such as body size, activity level, and medication. A general guideline is to fill about one-quarter to one-third of the plate with carbohydrate-rich foods. This approach helps prevent spikes in blood sugar levels post-meals.

Additionally, spreading carbohydrate intake evenly throughout the day can aid in maintaining a steadier glucose level, rather than consuming a large amount in one sitting.

Proteins: The Building Blocks

Proteins play a vital role in a diabetes-friendly diet, aiding in satiety, muscle repair, and overall metabolism. Unlike carbohydrates, proteins have a minimal impact on blood sugar levels, making them a crucial component of each meal. Sources of high-quality protein include lean meats, poultry, fish, tofu, legumes, and eggs. Incorporating protein into each meal and snack can help stabilize blood sugar levels by slowing the absorption of carbohydrates. It's not just the quantity but also the quality of protein that matters. Choosing lean protein sources and preparing them in healthy ways, such as grilling or baking rather than frying, can contribute to better diabetes management and overall health.

Fats: The Essential Moderators

Fats, though often misunderstood, are an essential part of a healthy diet, even for individuals with diabetes. They play a key role in nutrient absorption, hormone production, and brain function. The focus should be on the type of fat consumed. Monounsaturated and polyunsaturated fats, found in avocados, nuts, seeds, olive oil, and fatty fish like salmon, are heart-healthy choices. They can help improve blood cholesterol levels and reduce the risk of heart disease, a common complication of diabetes.

It's crucial to limit saturated fats and eliminate trans fats from the diet. These unhealthy fats, found in many fried foods, baked goods, and processed snacks, can raise bad cholesterol levels and increase the risk of heart disease. Balancing fat intake involves not only choosing healthy fats but also being mindful of portion sizes, as fats are calorie-dense.

The Balancing Act

Balancing carbohydrates, proteins, and fats in each meal can seem daunting, but it becomes more intuitive with practice. A practical approach is the plate method, where half the plate is filled with non-starchy vegetables, a quarter with lean protein, and the remaining quarter with complex carbohydrates. This visual guide simplifies meal planning and ensures a balance of nutrients.

Another aspect of this balance is understanding the glycemic impact of meals. Combining carbohydrates with proteins and fats can lower the overall glycemic effect, leading to more gradual increases in blood sugar levels. For instance, pairing a piece of fruit with a handful of nuts can provide a balanced snack that won't spike blood sugar levels.

Monitoring blood sugar responses to different food combinations can help fine-tune this balance. What works for one person may not work for another, making individual experimentation important. Consulting with a dietitian or diabetes educator can provide personalized guidance in finding the right balance.

Chapter 3: Preparing Your Kitchen for Success

Essential Kitchen Tools

Creating a kitchen environment conducive to successful diabetes management is akin to laying the foundation of a temple; it requires thought, care, and a selection of tools that resonate with the ethos of health and simplicity. The right tools in the kitchen can transform meal preparation from a daunting task into a seamless, enjoyable process, especially crucial for those managing Type 2 Diabetes.

The cornerstone of a well-equipped kitchen is a set of high-quality knives. A chef's knife, a paring knife, and a serrated knife form the triad that can tackle almost any cutting task. These knives must be kept sharp, as a sharp knife is safer and more efficient. The chef's knife, with its versatile blade, is ideal for chopping vegetables and herbs, crucial for diabetes-friendly diets rich in nutrients and fiber. The paring knife, smaller and more precise, is perfect for delicate tasks like peeling fruits or mincing garlic. The serrated knife, with its toothed edge, is the tool of choice for slicing bread or tomatoes without crushing them.

A set of sturdy cutting boards, preferably one for fresh produce and another for raw meats, is essential to maintain hygiene and prevent cross-contamination. Materials like bamboo or hard plastic are durable and less prone to harboring bacteria.

Measuring cups and spoons are indispensable in a kitchen where control over ingredients is vital. They ensure that recipes are followed accurately, an important aspect for meals that need to be balanced in nutrients and portion sizes. These tools help in maintaining the consistency of carbohydrate, protein, and fat intake, which is essential for blood sugar control.

A range of pots and pans is another pillar in the kitchen arsenal. A large skillet, a saucepan, and a stockpot cover most cooking needs. Non-stick cookware can be particularly helpful, as it requires less oil for cooking, aiding in preparing meals that are both healthy and flavorful.

An immersion blender or a traditional blender is a tool of convenience and versatility. It can be used for smoothies, soups, and sauces - all of which can be crafted to fit within a diabetes-friendly meal plan. The ability to quickly puree vegetables for soups or blend fruits for a nutritious smoothie makes meal preparation both simple and enjoyable.

A slow cooker or a pressure cooker is a boon for those with a busy lifestyle. These appliances allow for hands-off cooking, where meals can be prepared in bulk and with minimal effort. They are perfect for making stews, soups, and other one-pot meals that are nutrient-rich and can be portion-controlled easily.

Digital food scales are increasingly becoming a must-have tool in the modern kitchen. For someone with diabetes, knowing the exact weight of food helps in calculating carbohydrates and controlling portion sizes more accurately than volume measurements.

The spice rack, often overlooked, is a treasure trove of flavor. Herbs and spices are a way to add incredible flavor without adding extra carbohydrates or calories. Experimenting with different herbs and spices can turn a simple dish into a culinary delight, keeping meals interesting and appetizing.

Storage containers of various sizes aid in meal planning and portion control. They make it easy to store prepped ingredients, leftovers, and meal portions. Choosing containers that are freezer-safe and microwave-friendly adds to their convenience.

Lastly, a well-organized and accessible pantry and refrigerator are vital. Being able to easily find and reach for healthy ingredients encourages cooking at home and reduces the temptation of less healthy options.

Stocking Your Pantry

Stocking the pantry is a strategic endeavor in managing Type 2 Diabetes, much like a gardener carefully selects seeds for a bountiful harvest. The items on your shelves can either support or undermine your dietary goals, making it crucial to choose wisely and with foresight. A well-stocked pantry is the backbone of a kitchen where healthful and delicious meals are crafted, aligning with the nutritional needs of diabetes management.

Begin with whole grains, the stalwarts of a diabetes-friendly pantry. Quinoa, brown rice, barley, and whole wheat pasta offer complex carbohydrates, rich in fiber, which aid in regulating blood sugar levels and provide sustained energy. Their versatility allows them to be the foundation of many meals, from hearty breakfasts to satisfying dinners.

Legumes, including beans, lentils, and chickpeas, are champions in a diabetic diet. Packed with protein, fiber, and essential nutrients, they are a low-glycemic food choice that helps in stabilizing blood sugar. They can be incorporated into salads, soups, stews, or even as a meat substitute in various dishes.

Nuts and seeds are invaluable additions. Almonds, walnuts, chia seeds, and flaxseeds not only provide healthy fats but also add texture and flavor to meals. They can be sprinkled over salads, blended into smoothies, or simply enjoyed as a nutritious snack.

Stock a variety of canned goods, but choose wisely. Canned vegetables with no added salt, canned fruits in their own juice or light syrup, and low-sodium broths are convenient and can be life-savers in quick meal preparation. However, be mindful of the sodium and sugar content, which can be high in some canned products.

Herbs and spices are the essence of flavorful cooking without added sugar or salt. Basil, oregano, cinnamon, cumin, and turmeric not only enhance the taste of dishes but also offer health benefits, ranging from anti-inflammatory properties to blood sugar regulation.

Whole grain flours and meal options, like almond flour or oat flour, are better alternatives to refined white flour. They can be used in baking or as thickeners in sauces, providing more nutrients and less impact on blood sugar levels.

Oil is essential in cooking, but the type of oil matters. Olive oil, avocado oil, and other plant-based oils are preferable for their heart-healthy fats. They can be used for cooking, dressings, and marinades.

Vinegars and mustards, useful for dressings and marinades, add flavor without unwanted sugars or fats. Apple cider vinegar, balsamic vinegar, and Dijon mustard are versatile choices.

Sweeteners should be chosen with care. Stevia, erythritol, and other low-calorie sweeteners can be used in place of sugar. However, it's important to use them sparingly and be aware of how your body reacts to them.

Canned or jarred protein sources like tuna, salmon, or chicken can provide quick and easy protein for meals. Opt for versions with no added salt or packed in water.

In stocking your pantry, consider the shelf life and storage of items. Whole grains, for example, should be stored in airtight containers to maintain freshness. Regularly rotating stock and keeping an eye on expiration dates ensure that ingredients are fresh and nutritious.

Planning and Prepping Meals

Mastering the art of meal planning and preparation is a transformative practice for anyone, particularly for those managing Type 2 Diabetes. This process is akin to charting a course for a journey, ensuring that every step taken is in the right direction toward health and wellness. Meal planning and prepping not only aid in maintaining balanced blood sugar levels but also alleviate the daily stress of deciding what to eat, making healthy eating a practical and enjoyable part of life.

The journey of meal planning begins with mapping out meals for the week. This involves considering each meal and snack, ensuring they align with dietary goals. Planning should incorporate a variety of foods to provide balanced nutrition and prevent monotony. Include sources of complex carbohydrates, lean proteins, healthy fats, and plenty of vegetables. For each meal, visualize the plate, aiming for a harmonious balance of these components.

Once the plan is set, the next step is creating a shopping list. This list acts as a beacon, guiding you through the grocery store and helping you stay focused on purchasing nutritious ingredients while avoiding impulse buys that may not align with your dietary goals. Organize the list by sections of the store to make shopping more efficient and less overwhelming.

Prepping ingredients in advance is a cornerstone of meal planning. It involves washing, chopping, and sometimes cooking ingredients ahead of time. For instance, chopping vegetables for the week, cooking a batch of quinoa, or portioning out servings of nuts and seeds. These prepped ingredients become the building blocks for quick and easy meals throughout the week.

Cooking in bulk can save time and ensure that healthy options are always at hand. Preparing larger quantities of dishes like soups, stews, or casseroles allows for portions to be refrigerated or frozen for future meals. This strategy is particularly useful for busy days when cooking from scratch is less feasible.

Portion control is an essential aspect of meal prep, especially for individuals with diabetes. Pre-portioning meals can help manage carbohydrate intake and prevent overeating. Use measuring cups or a digital scale to ensure portions are consistent with your dietary plan.

Incorporate a day for experimentation and flexibility in your meal plan. This could be an opportunity to try new recipes or enjoy a meal out. It adds variety and enjoyment to the eating experience, making the diet more sustainable and less restrictive in the long run.

Labeling prepped meals and ingredients is a helpful practice. This not only helps in identifying the contents but also in tracking when they were prepared, ensuring food safety and freshness.

Be mindful of food safety when storing prepped ingredients. Most prepped vegetables, grains, and proteins will keep in the refrigerator for several days. Use airtight containers to preserve freshness and prevent contamination.

Regularly evaluate and adjust your meal planning and prepping routine. Consider what works well and what could be improved. This ongoing process allows you to refine your approach to better suit your lifestyle and dietary needs.

Finally, embrace the process with a positive mindset. Meal planning and prepping should not feel like a chore but rather an empowering practice that supports your health and well-being. It's a way to take control of your diet, ensuring that every meal is a step toward better diabetes management.

In conclusion, meal planning and prepping are about more than just organizing food; they are about setting the stage for healthier eating habits and taking control of diabetes management. This proactive approach helps in maintaining a balanced diet, reduces the stress of daily meal decisions, and supports overall health and wellness. With a thoughtful plan and prepared ingredients, each meal becomes an opportunity to nourish and sustain the body in the most healthful way possible.

Chapter 4: Breakfasts to Kickstart Your Day

Quick and Easy Options

Morning Zest Oat Bowl

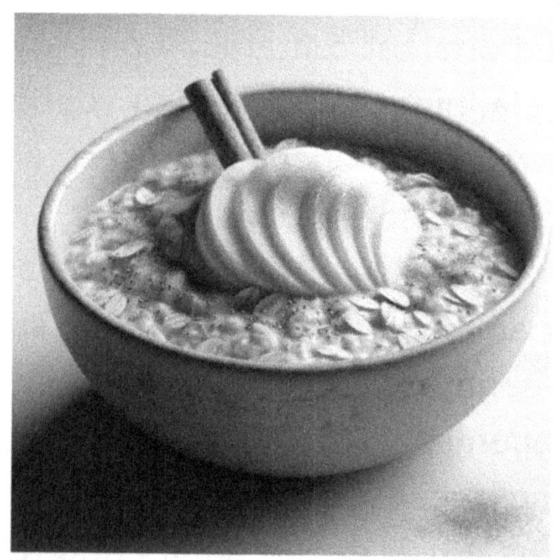

- **P.T.:** 10 mins
- **Ingr.:** Rolled oats (1/2 cup), unsweetened almond milk (1 cup), chia seeds (1 tbsp), grated apple (1/2), cinnamon (1/2 tsp)
- **Servings:** 1
- **Process:** Combine oats, almond milk, and chia seeds in a microwave-safe bowl. Microwave for 2-3 mins. Stir in grated apple and cinnamon.
- **Shopping List:** Rolled oats, unsweetened almond milk, chia seeds, apple, cinnamon.
- **Tips:** Soak oats and chia seeds overnight for a creamier texture.

<h1>Egg-Veggie Scramble</h1>

- **P.T.:** 15 mins
- **Ingr.:** Eggs (2), spinach (1 cup, chopped), cherry tomatoes (1/2 cup, halved), feta cheese (1/4 cup, crumbled), olive oil (1 tsp)
- **Servings:** 1
- **Process:** Heat olive oil in a skillet. Add spinach and tomatoes, sauté until wilted. Beat eggs and pour into skillet, stirring until cooked. Top with feta cheese.
- **Shopping List:** Eggs, spinach, cherry tomatoes, feta cheese, olive oil.
- **Tips:** Add a pinch of turmeric for extra flavor and health benefits.

<h1>Berry Yogurt Parfait</h1>

- **P.T.:** 10 mins
- **Ingr.:** Greek yogurt (1 cup, unsweetened), mixed berries (1/2 cup), almonds (2 tbsp, sliced), flaxseed meal (1 tbsp)
- **Servings:** 1
- **Process:** Layer yogurt, berries, and almonds in a glass. Sprinkle with flaxseed meal.
- **Shopping List:** Greek yogurt, mixed berries, almonds, flaxseed meal.
- **Tips:** Use frozen berries for a refreshing twist.

Avocado Toast Delight

- **P.T.:** 10 mins
- **Ingr.:** Whole grain bread (1 slice), ripe avocado (1/2, mashed), lemon juice (1 tsp), red pepper flakes (a pinch), sea salt (a pinch)
- **Servings:** 1
- **Process:** Toast bread until golden. Spread mashed avocado on toast, drizzle with lemon juice, and sprinkle with red pepper flakes and sea salt.
- **Shopping List:** Whole grain bread, avocado, lemon, red pepper flakes, sea salt.
- **Tips:** Add a poached egg on top for extra protein.

Smoothie Sunrise

- **P.T.:** 5 mins
- **Ingr.:** Spinach (1 cup), frozen mango (1/2 cup), unsweetened almond milk (1 cup), protein powder (1 scoop, optional), ginger (1/2 inch, grated)
- **Servings:** 1
- **Process:** Blend all ingredients until smooth.
- **Shopping List:** Spinach, frozen mango, unsweetened almond milk, protein powder, ginger.
- **Tips:** Add a tablespoon of chia seeds for extra fiber.

Cottage Cheese and Pineapple Bowl

- **P.T.:** 5 mins
- **Ingr.:** Cottage cheese (1/2 cup, low-fat), fresh pineapple (1/2 cup, diced), walnuts (1 tbsp, chopped), honey (1 tsp, optional)
- **Servings:** 1
- **Process:** Mix cottage cheese with pineapple. Top with walnuts and a drizzle of honey.
- **Shopping List:** Cottage cheese, fresh pineapple, walnuts, honey.
- **Tips:** Substitute pineapple with berries for a different flavor.

Power Seed Pudding

- **P.T.:** Overnight (prep), 5 mins (serving)
- **Ingr.:** Chia seeds (3 tbsp), unsweetened almond milk (1 cup), vanilla extract (1/2 tsp), mixed berries (1/2 cup)
- **Servings:** 1
- **Process:** Mix chia seeds, almond milk, and vanilla extract in a bowl. Refrigerate overnight. Serve topped with mixed berries.
- **Shopping List:** Chia seeds, unsweetened almond milk, vanilla extract, mixed berries.
- **Tips:** Stir the mixture a few times in the first hour of refrigeration to prevent clumping.

Weekend Specials

Savory Mediterranean Frittata

- **P.T.:** 25 mins
- **Ingr.:** Eggs (6), spinach (1 cup, chopped), cherry tomatoes (1/2 cup, halved), Kalamata olives (1/4 cup, pitted & sliced), feta cheese (1/3 cup, crumbled), olive oil (1 tbsp)
- **Servings:** 4
- **Process:** Whisk eggs. Sauté spinach and tomatoes in olive oil in an oven-safe skillet. Pour eggs over veggies, sprinkle olives and feta. Cook on stovetop for 5 mins, then bake at 375°F for 10 mins.
- **Shopping List:** Eggs, spinach, cherry tomatoes, Kalamata olives, feta cheese, olive oil.
- **Tips:** Add fresh herbs like basil or oregano for enhanced flavor.

Almond Flour Pancakes

- **P.T.:** 20 mins
- **Ingr.:** Almond flour (1 cup), eggs (2), unsweetened almond milk (1/2 cup), baking powder (1 tsp), vanilla extract (1 tsp), stevia (1 tbsp)
- **Servings:** 2-3
- **Process:** Mix all ingredients to form a batter. Pour scoops onto a greased skillet, cook until bubbles form, flip and cook until golden.
- **Shopping List:** Almond flour, eggs, unsweetened almond milk, baking powder, vanilla extract, stevia.
- **Tips:** Serve with a dollop of Greek yogurt and fresh berries.

Shakshuka Delight

- **P.T.:** 30 mins
- **Ingr.:** Eggs (4), canned tomatoes (1 can, diced), onion (1, diced), bell pepper (1, sliced), garlic (2 cloves, minced), cumin (1 tsp), paprika (1 tsp), olive oil (2 tbsp)
- **Servings:** 4
- **Process:** Sauté onion, bell pepper, and garlic in olive oil. Add tomatoes, cumin, paprika; simmer. Make wells, crack eggs into them. Cover, cook until eggs are set.
- **Shopping List:** Eggs, canned tomatoes, onion, bell pepper, garlic, cumin, paprika, olive oil.
- **Tips:** Garnish with cilantro and serve with whole grain toast.

Banana-Nut Oatmeal Bake

- **P.T.:** 35 mins
- **Ingr.:** Rolled oats (2 cups), ripe bananas (2, mashed), eggs (2), almond milk (1 cup), walnuts (1/2 cup, chopped), cinnamon (1 tsp), baking powder (1 tsp)
- **Servings:** 6
- **Process:** Mix all ingredients. Pour into a baking dish. Bake at 375°F for 25 mins.
- **Shopping List:** Rolled oats, bananas, eggs, almond milk, walnuts, cinnamon, baking powder.
- **Tips:** Drizzle with almond butter for extra richness.

Smoked Salmon Breakfast Wrap

- **P.T.:** 15 mins
- **Ingr.:** Whole grain tortillas (2), smoked salmon (4 oz), cream cheese (2 tbsp, light), capers (1 tbsp), red onion (1/4, thinly sliced), spinach leaves (1/2 cup)
- **Servings:** 2
- **Process:** Spread cream cheese on tortillas, add salmon, capers, onion, and spinach. Roll up tightly.
- **Shopping List:** Whole grain tortillas, smoked salmon, light cream cheese, capers, red onion, spinach.
- **Tips:** Add a squeeze of lemon juice for a zesty touch.

Mushroom and Spinach Breakfast Skillet

- **P.T.:** 25 mins
- **Ingr.:** Mushrooms (1 cup, sliced), spinach (2 cups), eggs (4), garlic (1 clove, minced), olive oil (1 tbsp), Parmesan cheese (2 tbsp, grated)
- **Servings:** 2
- **Process:** Sauté mushrooms and garlic in olive oil. Add spinach, cook until wilted. Crack eggs over, cover and cook until eggs are set. Sprinkle with Parmesan.
- **Shopping List:** Mushrooms, spinach, eggs, garlic, olive oil, Parmesan cheese.
- **Tips:** Serve with a side of salsa for a spicy kick.

Blueberry Almond Breakfast Quinoa

- **P.T.:** 20 mins
- **Ingr.:** Quinoa (1 cup, cooked), almond milk (1/2 cup), blueberries (1/2 cup), almonds (1/4 cup, sliced), cinnamon (1/2 tsp), stevia (1 tbsp)
- **Servings:** 2
- **Process:** Heat quinoa with almond milk, cinnamon, and stevia. Stir in blueberries and almonds before serving.
- **Shopping List:** Quinoa, almond milk, blueberries, almonds, cinnamon, stevia.
- **Tips:** Add a splash of vanilla extract for added flavor.

Breakfasts on the Go

Crispy Chickpea and Avocado Wrap

- **P.T.:** 15 mins
- **Ingr.:** Whole grain tortillas (2), canned chickpeas (1/2 cup, drained & rinsed), avocado (1, mashed), baby spinach (1 cup), lemon juice (1 tsp), smoked paprika (1/2 tsp)
- **Servings:** 2
- **Process:** Toss chickpeas with paprika. Spread mashed avocado on tortillas, top with chickpeas, spinach, and a drizzle of lemon juice. Roll up tightly.
- **Shopping List:** Whole grain tortillas, chickpeas, avocado, baby spinach, lemon, smoked paprika.
- **Tips:** Toast the wraps slightly for added crispness.

Apple-Cinnamon Overnight Oats

- **P.T.:** Overnight
- **Ingr.:** Rolled oats (1/2 cup), unsweetened almond milk (1/2 cup), apple (1, diced), chia seeds (1 tbsp), cinnamon (1/2 tsp), nutmeg (a pinch)
- **Servings:** 1
- **Process:** Mix all ingredients in a jar. Refrigerate overnight.
- **Shopping List:** Rolled oats, unsweetened almond milk, apple, chia seeds, cinnamon, nutmeg.
- **Tips:** Add a dollop of Greek yogurt for extra creaminess.

Berry Blast Smoothie

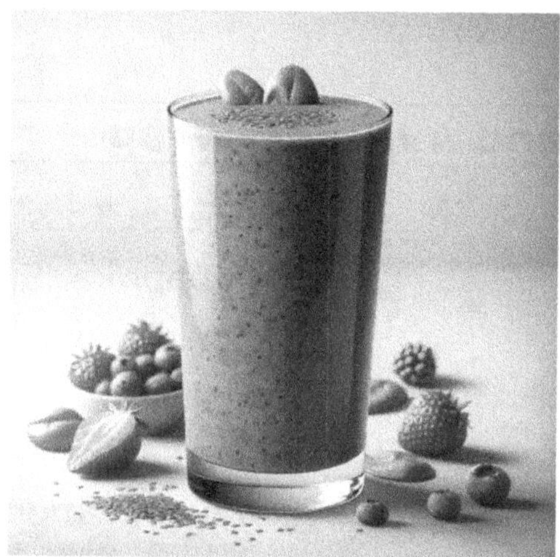

- **P.T.:** 5 mins
- **Ingr.:** Mixed berries (1 cup, frozen), spinach (1 cup), unsweetened almond milk (1 cup), flaxseed (1 tbsp), protein powder (1 scoop, optional)
- **Servings:** 1
- **Process:** Blend all ingredients until smooth.
- **Shopping List:** Mixed berries, spinach, unsweetened almond milk, flaxseed, protein powder.
- **Tips:** Add a tablespoon of almond butter for richness and healthy fats.

Veggie Hummus Pita Pocket

- **P.T.:** 10 mins
- **Ingr.:** Whole wheat pita bread (1), hummus (2 tbsp), cucumber (1/2, sliced), cherry tomatoes (1/2 cup, halved), arugula (1/2 cup)
- **Servings:** 1
- **Process:** Spread hummus inside pita. Fill with cucumber, tomatoes, and arugula.
- **Shopping List:** Whole wheat pita bread, hummus, cucumber, cherry tomatoes, arugula.
- **Tips:** Add sliced red onion for a flavor kick.

Almond Joy Yogurt Parfait

- **P.T.:** 10 mins
- **Ingr.:** Greek yogurt (1 cup, unsweetened), slivered almonds (2 tbsp), unsweetened coconut flakes (1 tbsp), dark chocolate chips (1 tbsp, sugar-free)
- **Servings:** 1
- **Process:** Layer yogurt with almonds, coconut flakes, and chocolate chips in a jar or bowl.
- **Shopping List:** Greek yogurt, slivered almonds, unsweetened coconut flakes, sugar-free dark chocolate chips.
- **Tips:** Layer the ingredients the night before for a quicker morning.

Spinach and Feta Breakfast Muffins

- **P.T.:** 30 mins
- **Ingr.:** Whole wheat flour (1 cup), eggs (3), feta cheese (1/2 cup, crumbled), spinach (1 cup, chopped), baking powder (1 tsp), olive oil (1 tbsp)
- **Servings:** 6 muffins
- **Process:** Mix eggs, feta, spinach, and olive oil. Add to flour and baking powder. Divide into muffin tins. Bake at 375°F for 20 mins.
- **Shopping List:** Whole wheat flour, eggs, feta cheese, spinach, baking powder, olive oil.
- **Tips:** Store in the fridge and reheat for a quick breakfast.

Peanut Butter and Banana Sandwich

- **P.T.:** 5 mins
- **Ingr.:** Whole grain bread (2 slices), natural peanut butter (2 tbsp), banana (1, sliced), cinnamon (a sprinkle)
- **Servings:** 1
- **Process:** Spread peanut butter on bread slices. Add banana slices and a sprinkle of cinnamon. Close sandwich.
- **Shopping List:** Whole grain bread, natural peanut butter, banana, cinnamon.
- **Tips:** Grill the sandwich for a warm, toasty breakfast.

Chapter 5: Light Bites and Snacks

Healthy Snacking

Spiced Roasted Chickpeas

- **P.T.:** 40 mins
- **Ingr.:** Chickpeas (1 can, drained & rinsed), olive oil (1 tbsp), cumin (1/2 tsp), smoked paprika (1/2 tsp), garlic powder (1/4 tsp)
- **Servings:** 4
- **Process:** Pat chickpeas dry, toss with oil and spices. Roast at 400°F for 30 mins, stirring halfway.
- **Shopping List:** Canned chickpeas, olive oil, cumin, smoked paprika, garlic powder.
- **Tips:** Let them cool completely for extra crunchiness.

Zucchini and Carrot Ribbon Salad

- **P.T.:** 15 mins
- **Ingr.:** Zucchini (1, large), carrot (1, large), lemon juice (2 tbsp), olive oil (1 tbsp), salt and pepper (to taste)
- **Servings:** 2
- **Process:** Use a peeler to create ribbons of zucchini and carrot. Toss with lemon juice, olive oil, salt, and pepper.
- **Shopping List:** Zucchini, carrot, lemon, olive oil.
- **Tips:** Add a sprinkle of chia seeds for an omega-3 boost.

Cucumber Hummus Bites

- **P.T.:** 10 mins
- **Ingr.:** Cucumber (1, sliced), hummus (1/2 cup), cherry tomatoes (1/4 cup, halved), Kalamata olives (1/4 cup, sliced)
- **Servings:** 4
- **Process:** Top cucumber slices with hummus, a tomato half, and an olive slice.
- **Shopping List:** Cucumber, hummus, cherry tomatoes, Kalamata olives.
- **Tips:** Garnish with fresh dill for added flavor.

Almond-Stuffed Dates

- **P.T.:** 10 mins
- **Ingr.:** Medjool dates (8), almonds (16), dark chocolate chips (1/4 cup, sugar-free), sea salt (a pinch)
- **Servings:** 4
- **Process:** Slit dates, remove pits. Insert an almond inside each date, press a chocolate chip on top, sprinkle with sea salt.
- **Shopping List:** Medjool dates, almonds, sugar-free dark chocolate chips, sea salt.
- **Tips:** Briefly warm in the microwave for a gooey treat.

Greek Yogurt and Berry Cups

- **P.T.:** 10 mins
- **Ingr.:** Greek yogurt (2 cups, unsweetened), mixed berries (1 cup), honey (2 tsp, optional), granola (1/4 cup, sugar-free)
- **Servings:** 4
- **Process:** Layer yogurt, berries, and granola in cups. Drizzle with honey.
- **Shopping List:** Greek yogurt, mixed berries, honey, sugar-free granola.
- **Tips:** Freeze for an hour for a frosty snack.

Avocado and Tomato Salad

- **P.T.:** 15 mins
- **Ingr.:** Avocado (1, diced), cherry tomatoes (1 cup, halved), red onion (1/4, finely chopped), cilantro (1/4 cup, chopped), lime juice (2 tbsp), salt and pepper (to taste)
- **Servings:** 2
- **Process:** Gently mix all ingredients in a bowl.
- **Shopping List:** Avocado, cherry tomatoes, red onion, cilantro, lime.
- **Tips:** Serve immediately to prevent avocado from browning.

Kale Chips with Nutritional Yeast

- **P.T.:** 20 mins
- **Ingr.:** Kale leaves (1 bunch, torn), olive oil (1 tbsp), nutritional yeast (2 tbsp), garlic powder (1/2 tsp), salt (1/4 tsp)
- **Servings:** 4
- **Process:** Toss kale with oil, nutritional yeast, garlic powder, and salt. Bake at 300°F for 15 mins, turning halfway.
- **Shopping List:** Kale, olive oil, nutritional yeast, garlic powder, salt.
- **Tips:** Ensure kale is dry before baking for optimal crispiness.

Dips and Spreads

Roasted Red Pepper Hummus

- **P.T.:** 15 mins
- **Ingr.:** Chickpeas (1 can, drained & rinsed), roasted red peppers (1/2 cup), tahini (2 tbsp), garlic (1 clove), lemon juice (2 tbsp), cumin (1/2 tsp)
- **Servings:** 4
- **Process:** Blend all ingredients until smooth. Add water if needed for consistency.
- **Shopping List:** Canned chickpeas, roasted red peppers, tahini, garlic, lemon, cumin.
- **Tips:** Garnish with chopped parsley and a drizzle of olive oil.

Avocado Greek Yogurt Dip

- **P.T.:** 10 mins
- **Ingr.:** Avocado (1, ripe), Greek yogurt (1/2 cup, unsweetened), lime juice (1 tbsp), garlic powder (1/2 tsp), cilantro (1/4 cup, chopped)
- **Servings:** 2-3
- **Process:** Mash avocado, mix with Greek yogurt, lime juice, garlic powder, and cilantro.
- **Shopping List:** Avocado, Greek yogurt, lime, garlic powder, cilantro.
- **Tips:** Chill for 30 mins before serving for enhanced flavors.

Sun-Dried Tomato Pesto

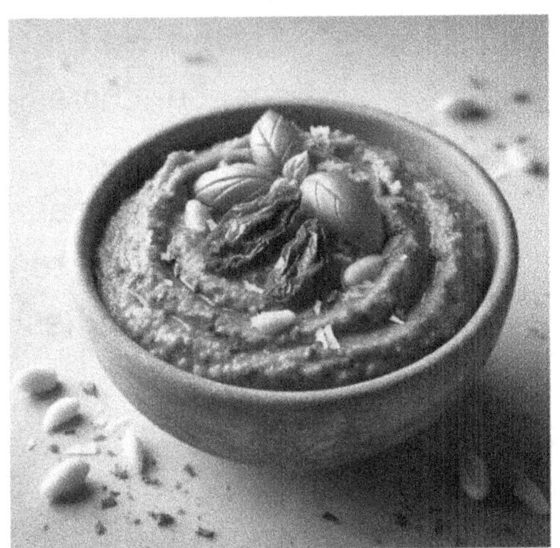

- **P.T.:** 10 mins
- **Ingr.:** Sun-dried tomatoes (1/2 cup), basil leaves (1 cup), pine nuts (1/4 cup), Parmesan cheese (1/4 cup, grated), olive oil (1/4 cup), garlic (1 clove)
- **Servings:** 4
- **Process:** Blend all ingredients until smooth, adding olive oil gradually.
- **Shopping List:** Sun-dried tomatoes, basil, pine nuts, Parmesan cheese, olive oil, garlic.
- **Tips:** Adjust garlic and basil to taste.

Spicy Black Bean Dip

- **P.T.:** 20 mins
- **Ingr.:** Black beans (1 can, drained & rinsed), jalapeño (1, seeded & chopped), lime juice (2 tbsp), cumin (1/2 tsp), cilantro (1/4 cup, chopped)
- **Servings:** 4
- **Process:** Blend beans, jalapeño, lime juice, and cumin until smooth. Stir in cilantro.
- **Shopping List:** Canned black beans, jalapeño, lime, cumin, cilantro.
- **Tips:** Serve with a dollop of Greek yogurt to balance the spice.

Herbed Cottage Cheese Spread

- **P.T.:** 10 mins
- **Ingr.:** Cottage cheese (1 cup, low-fat), chives (1/4 cup, chopped), dill (1 tbsp, chopped), lemon zest (1 tsp), black pepper (to taste)
- **Servings:** 2-3
- **Process:** Mix all ingredients until well combined.
- **Shopping List:** Cottage cheese, chives, dill, lemon, black pepper.
- **Tips:** Great as a spread on whole-grain toast or as a dip for veggies.

Baba Ganoush

- **P.T.:** 45 mins
- **Ingr.:** Eggplant (1 large), tahini (2 tbsp), garlic (2 cloves, minced), lemon juice (2 tbsp), olive oil (1 tbsp), smoked paprika (1/2 tsp)
- **Servings:** 4
- **Process:** Roast eggplant at 400°F for 30 mins. Scoop out flesh, blend with other ingredients.
- **Shopping List:** Eggplant, tahini, garlic, lemon, olive oil, smoked paprika.
- **Tips:** Add a pinch of cumin for an earthy flavor.

Creamy Walnut and Basil Spread

- **P.T.:** 15 mins
- **Ingr.:** Walnuts (1/2 cup, toasted), basil leaves (1 cup), Parmesan cheese (1/4 cup, grated), garlic (1 clove), olive oil (1/4 cup)
- **Servings:** 4
- **Process:** Blend walnuts, basil, Parmesan, and garlic, gradually add olive oil until creamy.
- **Shopping List:** Walnuts, basil, Parmesan cheese, garlic, olive oil.
- **Tips:** Perfect for spreading on cucumber slices or whole-grain crackers.

Sweet and Savory Treats

Cinnamon Spiced Nuts

- **P.T.:** 25 mins
- **Ingr.:** Mixed nuts (1 cup), egg white (1), cinnamon (1 tsp), stevia (1 tbsp), salt (a pinch)
- **Servings:** 4
- **Process:** Whisk egg white until frothy. Toss nuts in egg white, cinnamon, stevia, and salt. Bake at 300°F for 20 mins, stirring occasionally.
- **Shopping List:** Mixed nuts, egg white, cinnamon, stevia, salt.
- **Tips:** Let cool completely for added crunch.

Savory Roasted Chickpeas

- **P.T.:** 40 mins
- **Ingr.:** Chickpeas (1 can, drained & rinsed), olive oil (1 tbsp), garlic powder (1/2 tsp), smoked paprika (1/2 tsp), sea salt (1/4 tsp)
- **Servings:** 4
- **Process:** Toss chickpeas with oil and spices. Roast at 400°F for 30 mins.
- **Shopping List:** Canned chickpeas, olive oil, garlic powder, smoked paprika, sea salt.
- **Tips:** Roast until crispy for a satisfying snack.

Zucchini Parmesan Crisps

- **P.T.:** 30 mins
- **Ingr.:** Zucchini (2, thinly sliced), Parmesan cheese (1/2 cup, grated), olive oil (1 tbsp), black pepper (to taste)
- **Servings:** 4
- **Process:** Toss zucchini in olive oil, place on baking sheet, top with Parmesan and pepper. Bake at 375°F for 25 mins.
- **Shopping List:** Zucchini, Parmesan cheese, olive oil, black pepper.
- **Tips:** Slice zucchini evenly for consistent cooking.

Ricotta and Berry Tartlets

- **P.T.:** 20 mins
- **Ingr.:** Whole wheat mini tart shells (4), ricotta cheese (1/2 cup), mixed berries (1 cup), honey (1 tsp, optional), lemon zest (1 tsp)
- **Servings:** 4
- **Process:** Fill tart shells with ricotta, top with berries, drizzle with honey, and sprinkle lemon zest.
- **Shopping List:** Mini tart shells, ricotta cheese, mixed berries, honey, lemon.
- **Tips:** Use fresh berries for the best flavor and texture.

Spiced Pumpkin Seeds

- **P.T.:** 25 mins
- **Ingr.:** Pumpkin seeds (1 cup), olive oil (1 tbsp), chili powder (1/2 tsp), cumin (1/2 tsp), garlic powder (1/4 tsp), salt (to taste)
- **Servings:** 4
- **Process:** Toss seeds with oil and spices. Bake at 300°F for 20 mins, stirring occasionally.
- **Shopping List:** Pumpkin seeds, olive oil, chili powder, cumin, garlic powder, salt.
- **Tips:** Adjust spices to your preference.

Baked Apple Chips

- **P.T.:** 2 hrs
- **Ingr.:** Apples (2, thinly sliced), cinnamon (1 tsp), stevia (1 tbsp)
- **Servings:** 4
- **Process:** Arrange apple slices on a baking sheet, sprinkle with cinnamon and stevia. Bake at 200°F for 2 hrs, flipping halfway.
- **Shopping List:** Apples, cinnamon, stevia.
- **Tips:** Use a mandoline for evenly thin slices.

Mini Bell Pepper Nachos

- **P.T.:** 15 mins
- **Ingr.:** Mini bell peppers (1 cup, halved), black beans (1/2 cup, drained & rinsed), shredded cheese (1/2 cup, low-fat), avocado (1, diced), salsa (1/4 cup)
- **Servings:** 4
- **Process:** Arrange bell peppers on a baking sheet, top with black beans and cheese. Bake at 375°F for 10 mins. Top with avocado and salsa.
- **Shopping List:** Mini bell peppers, black beans, low-fat cheese, avocado, salsa.
- **Tips:** Add jalapeños for extra spice.

Chapter 6: Nutritious and Delicious Salads

Green and Leafy Varieties

Kale and Quinoa Power Salad

- **P.T.:** 20 mins
- **Ingr.:** Kale (2 cups, chopped), cooked quinoa (1 cup), cherry tomatoes (1/2 cup, halved), cucumber (1/2, diced), feta cheese (1/4 cup, crumbled), lemon vinaigrette (2 tbsp)
- **Servings:** 2
- **Process:** Toss kale, quinoa, tomatoes, cucumber, and feta. Drizzle with lemon vinaigrette.
- **Shopping List:** Kale, quinoa, cherry tomatoes, cucumber, feta cheese, lemon vinaigrette.
- **Tips:** Massage kale with a bit of olive oil to soften.

Spinach and Avocado Delight

- **P.T.:** 15 mins
- **Ingr.:** Spinach (2 cups), ripe avocado (1, sliced), red onion (1/4, thinly sliced), walnuts (1/4 cup, chopped), balsamic dressing (2 tbsp)
- **Servings:** 2
- **Process:** Combine spinach, avocado, onion, and walnuts. Toss with balsamic dressing.
- **Shopping List:** Spinach, avocado, red onion, walnuts, balsamic dressing.
- **Tips:** Add grilled chicken or tofu for extra protein.

Arugula and Pear Salad

- **P.T.:** 15 mins
- **Ingr.:** Arugula (2 cups), pear (1, thinly sliced), blue cheese (1/4 cup, crumbled), pecans (1/4 cup, toasted), honey mustard dressing (2 tbsp)
- **Servings:** 2
- **Process:** Mix arugula, pear slices, blue cheese, and pecans. Drizzle with honey mustard dressing.
- **Shopping List:** Arugula, pear, blue cheese, pecans, honey mustard dressing.
- **Tips:** Toast pecans in a dry pan for added flavor.

Minty Watermelon and Feta Salad

- **P.T.:** 20 mins
- **Ingr.:** Watermelon (2 cups, cubed), feta cheese (1/2 cup, crumbled), mint leaves (1/4 cup, chopped), black olives (1/4 cup, sliced), lime dressing (2 tbsp)
- **Servings:** 4
- **Process:** Combine watermelon, feta, mint, and olives. Toss with lime dressing.
- **Shopping List:** Watermelon, feta cheese, mint leaves, black olives, lime dressing.
- **Tips:** Chill the salad before serving for a refreshing taste.

Classic Caesar with a Twist

- **P.T.:** 20 mins
- **Ingr.:** Romaine lettuce (2 cups, chopped), grilled chicken strips (1 cup), Parmesan cheese (1/4 cup, shaved), whole grain croutons (1/2 cup), Caesar dressing (light, 2 tbsp)
- **Servings:** 2
- **Process:** Mix lettuce, chicken, Parmesan, and croutons. Add Caesar dressing and toss well.
- **Shopping List:** Romaine lettuce, grilled chicken, Parmesan cheese, whole grain croutons, light Caesar dressing.
- **Tips:** Swap chicken for grilled shrimp for variety.

Mixed Greens with Raspberry Vinaigrette

- **P.T.:** 15 mins
- **Ingr.:** Mixed greens (2 cups), raspberries (1/2 cup), goat cheese (1/4 cup, crumbled), almonds (1/4 cup, sliced), raspberry vinaigrette (2 tbsp)
- **Servings:** 2
- **Process:** Toss mixed greens with raspberries, goat cheese, and almonds. Drizzle with raspberry vinaigrette.
- **Shopping List:** Mixed greens, raspberries, goat cheese, almonds, raspberry vinaigrette.
- **Tips:** Add a sprinkle of chia seeds for extra nutrients.

Beet and Goat Cheese Salad

- **P.T.:** 30 mins
- **Ingr.:** Beets (2, roasted and sliced), mixed greens (2 cups), goat cheese (1/4 cup, crumbled), walnuts (1/4 cup, chopped), orange vinaigrette (2 tbsp)
- **Servings:** 2
- **Process:** Arrange beets over mixed greens. Top with goat cheese and walnuts. Drizzle with orange vinaigrette.
- **Shopping List:** Beets, mixed greens, goat cheese, walnuts, orange vinaigrette.
- **Tips:** Roast beets in advance to save time.

Protein-Packed Salads

Grilled Chicken and Avocado Salad

- **P.T.:** 25 mins
- **Ingr.:** Grilled chicken breast (1, sliced), mixed greens (2 cups), avocado (1, sliced), cherry tomatoes (1/2 cup, halved), red onion (1/4, thinly sliced), lemon vinaigrette (2 tbsp)
- **Servings:** 2
- **Process:** Arrange mixed greens on a plate, top with chicken, avocado, tomatoes, and onion. Drizzle with lemon vinaigrette.
- **Shopping List:** Chicken breast, mixed greens, avocado, cherry tomatoes, red onion, lemon vinaigrette.
- **Tips:** Marinate chicken in herbs and olive oil before grilling for added flavor.

Tuna and White Bean Salad

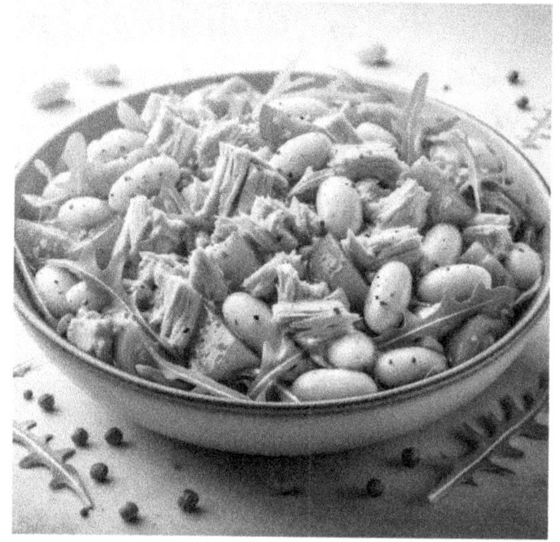

- **Servings:** 2
- **Process:** Mix tuna, beans, arugula, and bell pepper. Toss with vinaigrette.
- **Shopping List:** Canned tuna, white beans, arugula, red bell pepper, red wine vinaigrette.
- **Tips:** Add capers or olives for a Mediterranean twist.
- **P.T.:** 15 mins
- **Ingr.:** Canned tuna (1 can, drained), white beans (1 cup, rinsed & drained), arugula (2 cups), red bell pepper (1, diced), red wine vinaigrette (2 tbsp)

Egg and Spinach Cobb Salad

- **P.T.:** 20 mins
- **Ingr.:** Hard-boiled eggs (4, sliced), baby spinach (2 cups), cherry tomatoes (1/2 cup), avocado (1, diced), bacon (2 slices, cooked & crumbled), blue cheese dressing (2 tbsp)
- **Servings:** 2
- **Process:** Layer spinach, eggs, tomatoes, avocado, and bacon. Drizzle with dressing.
- **Shopping List:** Eggs, baby spinach, cherry tomatoes, avocado, bacon, blue cheese dressing.
- **Tips:** Swap bacon with turkey bacon for a healthier option.

Salmon and Asparagus Salad

- **P.T.:** 30 mins
- **Ingr.:** Grilled salmon fillet (1), asparagus (1 cup, blanched), mixed greens (2 cups), cucumber (1/2, sliced), dill vinaigrette (2 tbsp)
- **Servings:** 2
- **Process:** Place mixed greens on a plate, top with salmon, asparagus, and cucumber. Serve with dill vinaigrette.
- **Shopping List:** Salmon fillet, asparagus, mixed greens, cucumber, dill vinaigrette.
- **Tips:** Grill salmon with lemon and herbs for extra zest.

Turkey and Cranberry Spinach Salad

- **P.T.:** 15 mins
- **Ingr.:** Sliced turkey breast (1 cup), baby spinach (2 cups), dried cranberries (1/4 cup), walnuts (1/4 cup, chopped), balsamic vinaigrette (2 tbsp)
- **Servings:** 2
- **Process:** Combine spinach, turkey, cranberries, and walnuts. Toss with balsamic vinaigrette.
- **Shopping List:** Turkey breast, baby spinach, dried cranberries, walnuts, balsamic vinaigrette.
- **Tips:** Toast walnuts for added crunch and flavor.

Beef and Roasted Sweet Potato Salad

- **P.T.:** 35 mins
- **Ingr.:** Roast beef (1 cup, sliced), sweet potatoes (1 cup, cubed & roasted), arugula (2 cups), red onion (1/4, thinly sliced), mustard vinaigrette (2 tbsp)
- **Servings:** 2
- **Process:** Mix arugula, beef, sweet potatoes, and onion. Drizzle with mustard vinaigrette.
- **Shopping List:** Roast beef, sweet potatoes, arugula, red onion, mustard vinaigrette.
- **Tips:** Roast sweet potatoes with a sprinkle of cinnamon.

Quinoa and Black Bean Salad

- **P.T.:** 20 mins
- **Ingr.:** Cooked quinoa (1 cup), black beans (1 cup, rinsed & drained), corn (1/2 cup, cooked), cherry tomatoes (1/2 cup, halved), cilantro-lime dressing (2 tbsp)
- **Servings:** 2
- **Process:** Combine quinoa, beans, corn, and tomatoes. Toss with cilantro-lime dressing.
- **Shopping List:** Quinoa, black beans, corn, cherry tomatoes, cilantro-lime dressing.
- **Tips:** Add a diced avocado for creaminess and healthy fats.

Dressings and Vinaigrettes

Lemon Garlic Vinaigrette

- **P.T.:** 5 mins
- **Ingr.:** Olive oil (1/3 cup), lemon juice (3 tbsp), garlic (1 clove, minced), Dijon mustard (1 tsp), stevia (1/2 tsp), salt and pepper (to taste)
- **Servings:** 4-6
- **Process:** Whisk all ingredients until emulsified.
- **Shopping List:** Olive oil, lemon, garlic, Dijon mustard, stevia.
- **Tips:** Adjust garlic and lemon to suit your taste.

Creamy Avocado Dressing

- **P.T.:** 10 mins
- **Ingr.:** Ripe avocado (1), Greek yogurt (1/2 cup, unsweetened), lime juice (2 tbsp), cilantro (1/4 cup, chopped), garlic (1 clove), water (to thin), salt (to taste)
- **Servings:** 4
- **Process:** Blend all ingredients until smooth, adding water as needed for desired consistency.
- **Shopping List:** Avocado, Greek yogurt, lime, cilantro, garlic.
- **Tips:** Great as a dressing or a dip for veggies.

Balsamic and Maple Vinaigrette

- **P.T.:** 5 mins
- **Ingr.:** Balsamic vinegar (1/4 cup), olive oil (1/3 cup), maple syrup (1 tbsp, sugar-free), Dijon mustard (1 tsp), garlic powder (1/2 tsp), salt and pepper (to taste)
- **Servings:** 4-6
- **Process:** Shake or whisk all ingredients together.
- **Shopping List:** Balsamic vinegar, olive oil, sugar-free maple syrup, Dijon mustard, garlic powder.
- **Tips:** Store in the refrigerator for up to a week.

Cilantro Lime Dressing

- **P.T.:** 10 mins
- **Ingr.:** Cilantro (1 cup, packed), lime juice (3 tbsp), olive oil (1/4 cup), garlic (1 clove), honey (1 tsp, sugar-free), salt and pepper (to taste)
- **Servings:** 4
- **Process:** Blend all ingredients until smooth.
- **Shopping List:** Cilantro, lime, olive oil, garlic, sugar-free honey.
- **Tips:** Adjust cilantro and lime ratio to get the right zing.

Ginger Sesame Dressing

- **P.T.:** 10 mins
- **Ingr.:** Sesame oil (1/4 cup), rice vinegar (1/4 cup), soy sauce (low sodium, 2 tbsp), ginger (1 tbsp, grated), garlic (1 clove, minced), stevia (1 tsp)
- **Servings:** 4
- **Process:** Whisk together all ingredients until well combined.
- **Shopping List:** Sesame oil, rice vinegar, low sodium soy sauce, ginger, garlic, stevia.
- **Tips:** Perfect for Asian-style salads or as a marinade.

Honey Mustard Vinaigrette

- **P.T.:** 5 mins
- **Ingr.:** Olive oil (1/3 cup), apple cider vinegar (2 tbsp), Dijon mustard (1 tbsp), honey (1 tbsp, sugar-free), garlic powder (1/2 tsp), salt and pepper (to taste)
- **Servings:** 4-6
- **Process:** Combine all ingredients and shake well.
- **Shopping List:** Olive oil, apple cider vinegar, Dijon mustard, sugar-free honey, garlic powder.
- **Tips:** Adjust the amount of honey and mustard to balance sweetness and tanginess.

Raspberry Walnut Vinaigrette

- **P.T.:** 10 mins
- **Ingr.:** Raspberry vinegar (1/4 cup), olive oil (1/3 cup), walnut oil (1 tbsp), stevia (1 tsp), salt and pepper (to taste)
- **Servings:** 4-6
- **Process:** Whisk all ingredients together until emulsified.
- **Shopping List:** Raspberry vinegar, olive oil, walnut oil, stevia.
- **Tips:** Drizzle over a spinach and goat cheese salad for a delightful pairing.

Chapter 7: Soups and Stews for the Soul

Comforting Soups

Turmeric Chicken Soup

- **P.T.:** 35 mins
- **Ingr.:** Chicken breast (1, diced), carrots (2, chopped), celery (2 stalks, chopped), onion (1, diced), garlic (2 cloves, minced), turmeric (1 tsp), chicken broth (4 cups, low sodium), spinach (1 cup), olive oil (1 tbsp)
- **Servings:** 4
- **Process:** Sauté onion, garlic, carrots, and celery in olive oil. Add chicken, turmeric, and broth. Simmer until chicken is cooked. Stir in spinach before serving.
- **Shopping List:** Chicken breast, carrots, celery, onion, garlic, turmeric, chicken broth, spinach, olive oil.
- **Tips:** Add ginger for an extra immune boost.

Lentil and Vegetable Soup

- **P.T.:** 45 mins
- **Ingr.:** Lentils (1 cup), diced tomatoes (1 can), carrots (2, chopped), celery (2 stalks, chopped), onion (1, diced), vegetable broth (4 cups), thyme (1 tsp), olive oil (1 tbsp)
- **Servings:** 4-6
- **Process:** Cook onion, carrots, and celery in olive oil. Add lentils, tomatoes, broth, and thyme. Simmer until lentils are tender.
- **Shopping List:** Lentils, canned tomatoes, carrots, celery, onion, vegetable broth, thyme, olive oil.
- **Tips:** Soak lentils beforehand to reduce cooking time.

Hearty Beef and Barley Soup

- **P.T.:** 1 hr
- **Ingr.:** Beef stew meat (1 lb), barley (1/2 cup), beef broth (4 cups, low sodium), carrots (2, chopped), onion (1, chopped), celery (2 stalks, chopped), olive oil (1 tbsp), Worcestershire sauce (1 tbsp)
- **Servings:** 4

- **Process:** Brown beef in olive oil. Add vegetables, barley, broth, and Worcestershire sauce. Simmer until barley and beef are tender.
- **Shopping List:** Beef stew meat, barley, beef broth, carrots, onion, celery, olive oil, Worcestershire sauce.
- **Tips:** Skim off any fat that rises to the top for a healthier soup.

Creamy Cauliflower Soup

- **P.T.:** 30 mins
- **Ingr.:** Cauliflower (1 head, chopped), garlic (3 cloves, minced), onion (1, diced), vegetable broth (4 cups), almond milk (1 cup), nutmeg (a pinch), olive oil (1 tbsp)
- **Servings:** 4

- **Process:** Sauté onion and garlic in oil. Add cauliflower, broth, and nutmeg. Simmer until soft, blend until smooth. Stir in almond milk.
- **Shopping List:** Cauliflower, garlic, onion, vegetable broth, almond milk, nutmeg, olive oil.
- **Tips:** Garnish with roasted cauliflower florets.

Spicy Tomato and Chickpea Soup

- **P.T.:** 30 mins
- **Ingr.:** Chickpeas (1 can, drained & rinsed), diced tomatoes (1 can), onion (1, diced), garlic (2 cloves, minced), cumin (1 tsp), chili powder (1/2 tsp), vegetable broth (4 cups), olive oil (1 tbsp)
- **Servings:** 4
- **Process:** Cook onion and garlic in olive oil. Add spices, chickpeas, tomatoes, and broth. Simmer for 20 mins.
- **Shopping List:** Canned chickpeas, canned tomatoes, onion, garlic, cumin, chili powder, vegetable broth, olive oil.
- **Tips:** Add a dollop of Greek yogurt to balance the spice.

Mushroom and Wild Rice Soup

- **P.T.:** 50 mins
- **Ingr.:** Wild rice (1/2 cup), assorted mushrooms (2 cups, sliced), onion (1, diced), garlic (2 cloves, minced), thyme (1 tsp), vegetable broth (4 cups), cream (1/4 cup, optional), olive oil (1 tbsp)
- **Servings:** 4
- **Process:** Sauté mushrooms, onion, and garlic in oil. Add rice, thyme, and broth. Simmer until rice is cooked. Stir in cream if using.
- **Shopping List:** Wild rice, mushrooms, onion, garlic, thyme, vegetable broth, cream, olive oil.
- **Tips:** Toast the rice slightly before adding broth for added flavor.

Butternut Squash and Ginger Soup

- **P.T.:** 45 mins
- **Ingr.:** Butternut squash (1, peeled & cubed), ginger (1 tbsp, grated), onion (1, diced), vegetable broth (4 cups), coconut milk (1 cup), curry powder (1 tsp), olive oil (1 tbsp)
- **Servings:** 4
- **Process:** Cook onion and ginger in oil. Add squash, curry, and broth. Simmer until soft. Blend until smooth, add coconut milk.
- **Shopping List:** Butternut squash, ginger, onion, vegetable broth, coconut milk, curry powder, olive oil.
- **Tips:** Serve with a sprinkle of roasted pumpkin seeds.

Hearty Stews

White Bean and Kale Stew

- **P.T.:** 40 mins
- **Ingr.:** White beans (1 can, drained & rinsed), kale (2 cups, chopped), carrots (2, diced), onion (1, diced), garlic (2 cloves, minced), vegetable broth (4 cups), thyme (1 tsp), olive oil (1 tbsp)
- **Servings:** 4
- **Process:** Sauté onion, garlic, and carrots in olive oil. Add beans, kale, thyme, and broth. Simmer until vegetables are tender.
- **Shopping List:** White beans, kale, carrots, onion, garlic, vegetable broth, thyme, olive oil.
- **Tips:** Serve with a sprinkle of Parmesan cheese for added flavor.

Beef and Vegetable Stew

- **P.T.:** 1 hr 20 mins
- **Ingr.:** Beef stew meat (1 lb), mixed vegetables (2 cups, chopped), beef broth (4 cups), tomato paste (2 tbsp), Worcestershire sauce (1 tbsp), bay leaf (1), olive oil (1 tbsp)
- **Servings:** 4
- **Process:** Brown beef in olive oil. Add vegetables, broth, tomato paste, Worcestershire sauce, and bay leaf. Simmer until meat is tender.
- **Shopping List:** Beef stew meat, mixed vegetables, beef broth, tomato paste, Worcestershire sauce, bay leaf, olive oil.
- **Tips:** Thicken the stew with a little cornstarch if desired.

Chicken and Lentil Soup

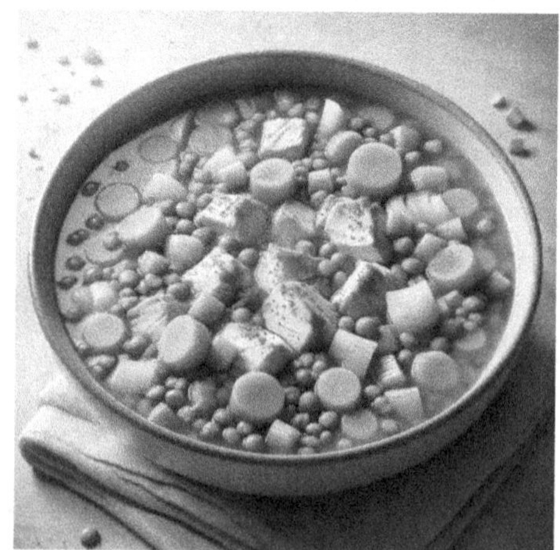

- **P.T.:** 50 mins
- **Ingr.:** Chicken breast (1 lb, diced), lentils (1 cup), onion (1, diced), carrots (2, diced), celery (2 stalks, diced), chicken broth (4 cups), cumin (1 tsp), olive oil (1 tbsp)
- **Servings:** 4
- **Process:** Cook chicken, onion, carrots, and celery in olive oil. Add lentils, cumin, and broth. Simmer until lentils are tender.
- **Shopping List:** Chicken breast, lentils, onion, carrots, celery, chicken broth, cumin, olive oil.
- **Tips:** Add a squeeze of lemon juice for a fresh flavor.

Moroccan Chickpea Stew

- **P.T.:** 45 mins
- **Ingr.:** Chickpeas (1 can, drained & rinsed), diced tomatoes (1 can), onion (1, diced), garlic (2 cloves, minced), spinach (2 cups), cumin (1 tsp), cinnamon (1/2 tsp), vegetable broth (4 cups), olive oil (1 tbsp)
- **Servings:** 4
- **Process:** Sauté onion and garlic in olive oil. Add spices, chickpeas, tomatoes, and broth. Simmer for 30 mins. Stir in spinach before serving.
- **Shopping List:** Chickpeas, diced tomatoes, onion, garlic, spinach, cumin, cinnamon, vegetable broth, olive oil.
- **Tips:** Top with fresh cilantro and a dollop of Greek yogurt.

Squash and Turkey Chili

- **P.T.:** 1 hr
- **Ingr.:** Ground turkey (1 lb), butternut squash (2 cups, cubed), onion (1, diced), bell pepper (1, diced), canned tomatoes (1 can), chili powder (1 tbsp), cumin (1 tsp), chicken broth (3 cups)
- **Servings:** 4
- **Process:** Brown turkey with onion and bell pepper. Add squash, tomatoes, spices, and broth. Simmer until squash is tender.
- **Shopping List:** Ground turkey, butternut squash, onion, bell pepper, canned tomatoes, chili powder, cumin, chicken broth.
- **Tips:** Serve with a sprinkle of shredded cheese and avocado slices.

Italian Sausage and Bean Soup

- **P.T.:** 45 mins
- **Ingr.:** Italian sausage (1 lb, sliced), cannellini beans (1 can, drained & rinsed), kale (2 cups, chopped), onion (1, diced), garlic (2 cloves, minced), chicken broth (4 cups), Italian seasoning (1 tsp), olive oil (1 tbsp)
- **Servings:** 4
- **Process:** Cook sausage, onion, and garlic in olive oil. Add beans, kale, seasoning, and broth. Simmer until kale is wilted.
- **Shopping List:** Italian sausage, cannellini beans, kale, onion, garlic, chicken broth, Italian seasoning, olive oil.
- **Tips:** Add red pepper flakes for extra heat.

Miso Vegetable Stew

- **P.T.:** 35 mins
- **Ingr.:** Miso paste (2 tbsp), tofu (1 cup, cubed), mixed vegetables (2 cups, chopped), shiitake mushrooms (1 cup, sliced), seaweed (1/4 cup, chopped), vegetable broth (4 cups), ginger (1 tbsp, grated)
- **Servings:** 4
- **Process:** Dissolve miso in broth, add ginger, tofu, vegetables, and mushrooms. Simmer gently, do not boil. Add seaweed before serving.
- **Shopping List:** Miso paste, tofu, mixed vegetables, shiitake mushrooms, seaweed, vegetable broth, ginger.
- **Tips:** Adjust miso quantity to taste, as it's quite salty.

Chilled Soups for Summer

Gazpacho Andaluz

- **P.T.:** 20 mins (plus chilling)
- **Ingr.:** Ripe tomatoes (4, large, chopped), cucumber (1, peeled & chopped), bell pepper (1, chopped), red onion (1/2, chopped), garlic (1 clove), red wine vinegar (2 tbsp), olive oil (2 tbsp), salt and pepper (to taste)
- **Servings:** 4
- **Process:** Blend all ingredients until smooth. Chill for at least 2 hours before serving.
- **Shopping List:** Ripe tomatoes, cucumber, bell pepper, red onion, garlic, red wine vinegar, olive oil.
- **Tips:** Serve with a sprinkle of chopped herbs and croutons.

Chilled Cucumber Avocado Soup

- **P.T.:** 15 mins (plus chilling)
- **Ingr.:** Cucumbers (2, large, peeled & chopped), avocado (1, ripe), yogurt (1 cup, plain, unsweetened), lemon juice (2 tbsp), garlic (1 clove), dill (1 tbsp, fresh), salt and pepper (to taste)
- **Servings:** 4
- **Process:** Puree cucumbers, avocado, yogurt, lemon juice, garlic, and dill until smooth. Season and chill.
- **Shopping List:** Cucumbers, avocado, plain yogurt, lemon, garlic, dill.
- **Tips:** Add a dash of hot sauce for a spicy kick.

Melon and Mint Soup

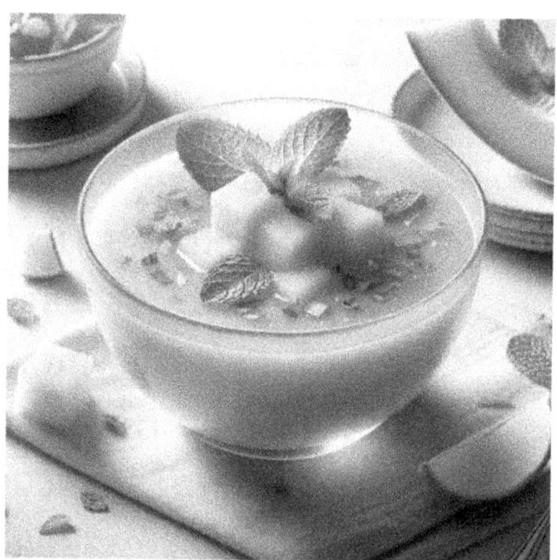

- **P.T.:** 15 mins (plus chilling)
- **Ingr.:** Cantaloupe (1, cubed), lime juice (3 tbsp), honey (1 tbsp, sugar-free), fresh mint (1/4 cup, chopped), ginger (1 tsp, grated)
- **Servings:** 4
- **Process:** Blend melon, lime juice, honey, mint, and ginger. Chill thoroughly.
- **Shopping List:** Cantaloupe, lime, sugar-free honey, fresh mint, ginger.
- **Tips:** Garnish with extra mint and lime zest.

Beetroot and Yogurt Soup

- **P.T.:** 30 mins (plus chilling)
- **Ingr.:** Cooked beets (2 cups, diced), Greek yogurt (1 cup, unsweetened), cucumber (1, diced), dill (1 tbsp, chopped), garlic (1 clove), lemon juice (2 tbsp)
- **Servings:** 4
- **Process:** Puree beets, yogurt, cucumber, dill, garlic, and lemon juice. Season and chill.
- **Shopping List:** Cooked beets, Greek yogurt, cucumber, dill, garlic, lemon.
- **Tips:** Serve with a swirl of yogurt and a sprinkle of dill.

Pea and Mint Soup

- **P.T.:** 20 mins (plus chilling)
- **Ingr.:** Green peas (2 cups, fresh or frozen), vegetable broth (3 cups), mint leaves (1/4 cup), onion (1, diced), garlic (1 clove), olive oil (1 tbsp), lemon juice (1 tbsp)
- **Servings:** 4
- **Process:** Sauté onion and garlic in olive oil. Add peas, broth, and mint. Simmer, blend, then chill.
- **Shopping List:** Green peas, vegetable broth, mint leaves, onion, garlic, olive oil, lemon.
- **Tips:** Add a dollop of yogurt when serving for creaminess.

Tomato and Basil Soup

- **P.T.:** 30 mins (plus chilling)
- **Ingr.:** Ripe tomatoes (6, large, chopped), basil leaves (1/2 cup), vegetable broth (3 cups), garlic (2 cloves), onion (1, diced), olive oil (1 tbsp), balsamic vinegar (1 tbsp)
- **Servings:** 4
- **Process:** Cook onion and garlic in olive oil. Add tomatoes, broth, and basil. Simmer, blend, then chill.
- **Shopping List:** Ripe tomatoes, basil leaves, vegetable broth, garlic, onion, olive oil, balsamic vinegar.
- **Tips:** Garnish with fresh basil and a drizzle of olive oil.

Carrot Ginger Soup

- **P.T.:** 30 mins (plus chilling)
- **Ingr.:** Carrots (4, large, chopped), ginger (2 tbsp, grated), orange juice (1/2 cup), vegetable broth (4 cups), onion (1, diced), garlic (1 clove), olive oil (1 tbsp)
- **Servings:** 4
- **Process:** Sauté onion, garlic, and ginger in oil. Add carrots, broth, and orange juice. Simmer, blend, then chill.
- **Shopping List:** Carrots, ginger, orange juice, vegetable broth, onion, garlic, olive oil.
- **Tips:** Serve with a swirl of cream for added richness.

Chapter 8: Main Course Magic

Vegetarian Delights

Eggplant Parmesan Stack

- **P.T.:** 50 mins
- **Ingr.:** Eggplant (1, sliced), marinara sauce (2 cups), mozzarella cheese (1 cup, shredded), Parmesan cheese (1/2 cup, grated), basil leaves (1/4 cup), olive oil (for brushing)
- **Servings:** 4
- **Process:** Brush eggplant slices with oil, bake at 375°F for 25 mins. Layer eggplant, marinara, mozzarella, and basil. Bake for 20 more mins.
- **Shopping List:** Eggplant, marinara sauce, mozzarella cheese, Parmesan cheese, basil, olive oil.
- **Tips:** Let the eggplant sit with salt for 30 mins before cooking to remove bitterness.

Chickpea and Spinach Curry

- **P.T.:** 35 mins
- **Ingr.:** Chickpeas (1 can, drained & rinsed), spinach (2 cups), onion (1, diced), garlic (2 cloves, minced), curry powder (1 tbsp), coconut milk (1 can), olive oil (1 tbsp)
- **Servings:** 4
- **Process:** Sauté onion and garlic in oil. Add curry powder, chickpeas, and coconut milk. Simmer for 15 mins. Stir in spinach until wilted.
- **Shopping List:** Chickpeas, spinach, onion, garlic, curry powder, coconut milk, olive oil.
- **Tips:** Serve with cauliflower rice for a low-carb option.

Zucchini Lasagna Rolls

- **P.T.:** 45 mins
- **Ingr.:** Zucchini (4, sliced lengthwise), ricotta cheese (1 cup), spinach (1 cup, chopped), marinara sauce (2 cups), mozzarella cheese (1/2 cup, shredded), egg (1), garlic (1 clove, minced)
- **Servings:** 4
- **Process:** Mix ricotta, spinach, egg, and garlic. Spread on zucchini slices, roll up, place in baking dish. Top with sauce and mozzarella. Bake at 375°F for 25 mins.
- **Shopping List:** Zucchini, ricotta cheese, spinach, marinara sauce, mozzarella cheese, egg, garlic.
- **Tips:** Grill zucchini slices briefly before rolling for better texture.

Stuffed Bell Peppers with Quinoa

- **P.T.:** 1 hr
- **Ingr.:** Bell peppers (4, halved and seeded), cooked quinoa (2 cups), black beans (1 can, drained & rinsed), corn (1 cup), tomato sauce (1 cup), cumin (1 tsp), cheese (1/2 cup, shredded)
- **Servings:** 4
- **Process:** Mix quinoa, beans, corn, tomato sauce, and cumin. Stuff peppers, top with cheese. Bake at 350°F for 30 mins.
- **Shopping List:** Bell peppers, quinoa, black beans, corn, tomato sauce, cumin, cheese.
- **Tips:** Add chopped jalapeños to the filling for a spicy kick.

Vegetable Stir-Fry with Tofu

- **P.T.:** 30 mins
- **Ingr.:** Tofu (1 block, pressed & cubed), assorted vegetables (3 cups, chopped), soy sauce (low sodium, 2 tbsp), ginger (1 tbsp, grated), garlic (2 cloves, minced), sesame oil (1 tbsp), olive oil (1 tbsp)
- **Servings:** 4
- **Process:** Sauté tofu in olive oil until golden. Remove. Cook vegetables, ginger, and garlic in sesame oil. Add tofu and soy sauce. Stir well.
- **Shopping List:** Tofu, assorted vegetables, low sodium soy sauce, ginger, garlic, sesame oil, olive oil.
- **Tips:** Marinate tofu in soy sauce and ginger before cooking for more flavor.

Portobello Mushroom Fajitas

- **P.T.:** 25 mins
- **Ingr.:** Portobello mushrooms (4, sliced), bell peppers (2, sliced), onion (1, sliced), fajita seasoning (1 tbsp), olive oil (2 tbsp), whole wheat tortillas (4)
- **Servings:** 4
- **Process:** Sauté mushrooms, peppers, and onion with seasoning in oil. Serve on tortillas.
- **Shopping List:** Portobello mushrooms, bell peppers, onion, fajita seasoning, olive oil, whole wheat tortillas.
- **Tips:** Add avocado slices for creaminess and healthy fats.

Lentil Sloppy Joes

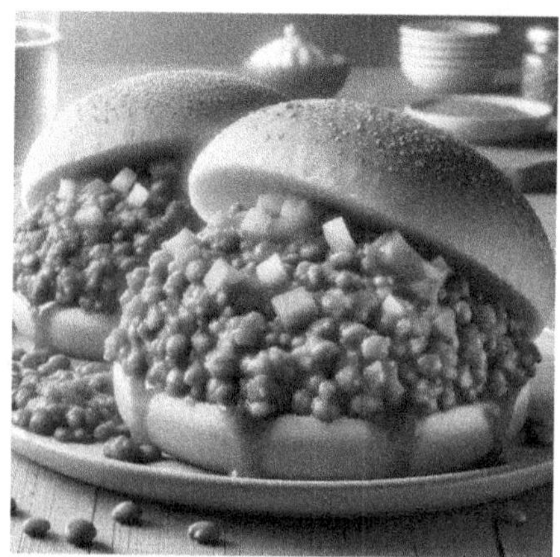

- **P.T.:** 45 mins
- **Ingr.:** Lentils (1 cup, cooked), onion (1, diced), garlic (2 cloves, minced), bell pepper (1, diced), tomato sauce (1 cup), maple syrup (1 tbsp, sugar-free), whole wheat buns (4)
- **Servings:** 4
- **Process:** Cook onion, garlic, and bell pepper. Add lentils, tomato sauce, and maple syrup. Simmer for 20 mins. Serve on buns.
- **Shopping List:** Lentils, onion, garlic, bell pepper, tomato sauce, sugar-free maple syrup, whole wheat buns.
- **Tips:** Add a splash of Worcestershire sauce for depth of flavor.

Meat and Poultry Favorites

Herb-Crusted Chicken Breast

- **P.T.:** 30 mins
- **Ingr.:** Chicken breasts (4, boneless), mixed herbs (2 tbsp, chopped, e.g., rosemary, thyme), garlic (2 cloves, minced), lemon zest (1 tsp), olive oil (2 tbsp), salt and pepper (to taste)
- **Servings:** 4
- **Process:** Combine herbs, garlic, lemon zest, salt, pepper, and olive oil. Rub on chicken. Bake at 375°F for 25 mins.
- **Shopping List:** Chicken breasts, mixed herbs, garlic, lemon, olive oil.
- **Tips:** Let chicken rest for 5 mins before serving for juiciness.

Balsamic Glazed Pork Chops

- **P.T.:** 25 mins
- **Ingr.:** Pork chops (4, bone-in), balsamic vinegar (1/4 cup), garlic (2 cloves, minced), honey (1 tbsp, sugar-free), olive oil (1 tbsp), rosemary (1 tsp, chopped), salt and pepper (to taste)
- **Servings:** 4
- **Process:** Sauté pork chops in olive oil. Mix vinegar, garlic, honey, and rosemary. Pour over chops, simmer until cooked.
- **Shopping List:** Pork chops, balsamic vinegar, garlic, sugar-free honey, olive oil, rosemary.
- **Tips:** Marinate chops for an hour in the fridge for deeper flavor.

Turkey Meatloaf with Sun-Dried Tomatoes

- **P.T.:** 1 hr 10 mins
- **Ingr.:** Ground turkey (1 lb), sun-dried tomatoes (1/2 cup, chopped), onion (1, diced), garlic (2 cloves, minced), egg (1), whole wheat breadcrumbs (1/2 cup), Italian seasoning (1 tbsp), tomato paste (for topping, 2 tbsp)
- **Servings:** 4
- **Process:** Mix all ingredients except tomato paste. Form into a loaf, top with tomato paste. Bake at 375°F for 50 mins.
- **Shopping List:** Ground turkey, sun-dried tomatoes, onion, garlic, egg, whole wheat breadcrumbs, Italian seasoning, tomato paste.
- **Tips:** Let meatloaf rest for 10 mins before slicing.

Beef and Broccoli Stir-Fry

- **P.T.:** 30 mins
- **Ingr.:** Beef strips (1 lb), broccoli (2 cups, florets), soy sauce (low sodium, 3 tbsp), ginger (1 tbsp, grated), garlic (2 cloves, minced), sesame oil (1 tbsp), olive oil (1 tbsp)
- **Servings:** 4
- **Process:** Stir-fry beef in olive oil, set aside. Cook broccoli in sesame oil, add ginger, garlic. Add beef, soy sauce. Stir well.
- **Shopping List:** Beef strips, broccoli, low sodium soy sauce, ginger, garlic, sesame oil, olive oil.
- **Tips:** Marinate beef in soy sauce and ginger for at least 30 mins.

Lemon Thyme Roast Chicken

- **P.T.:** 1 hr 20 mins
- **Ingr.:** Whole chicken (1, 4 lbs), lemon (1, sliced), thyme (1 bunch), garlic (4 cloves), butter (2 tbsp, unsalted), salt and pepper (to taste)
- **Servings:** 4-6
- **Process:** Stuff chicken with lemon, thyme, and garlic. Rub butter on skin, season. Roast at 375°F for 1 hr 10 mins.
- **Shopping List:** Whole chicken, lemon, thyme, garlic, butter.
- **Tips:** Let chicken rest before carving for better flavor distribution.

Spiced Lamb Kebabs

- **P.T.:** 45 mins (plus marinating time)
- **Ingr.:** Lamb (1 lb, cubed), yogurt (1/2 cup, plain), cumin (1 tsp), coriander (1 tsp), garlic (2 cloves, minced), lemon juice (2 tbsp), salt and pepper (to taste)
- **Servings:** 4
- **Process:** Marinate lamb in yogurt, spices, garlic, lemon juice. Skewer and grill for 10-15 mins.
- **Shopping List:** Lamb, yogurt, cumin, coriander, garlic, lemon.
- **Tips:** Serve with a side of cucumber yogurt sauce.

Chicken Fajitas with Bell Peppers

- **P.T.:** 35 mins
- **Ingr.:** Chicken breast (2, sliced), bell peppers (3, assorted colors, sliced), onion (1, sliced), fajita seasoning (2 tbsp), olive oil (2 tbsp), whole wheat tortillas (4)
- **Servings:** 4
- **Process:** Sauté chicken in 1 tbsp oil, set aside. Cook peppers and onion in remaining oil. Add chicken, seasoning. Serve with tortillas.
- **Shopping List:** Chicken breast, bell peppers, onion, fajita seasoning, olive oil, whole wheat tortillas.
- **Tips:** Add lime juice and cilantro for extra freshness.

Fish and Seafood Specials

Grilled Salmon with Herb Rub

- **P.T.:** 25 mins
- **Ingr.:** Salmon fillets (4), olive oil (2 tbsp), lemon zest (1 tsp), dill (1 tbsp, chopped), garlic (1 clove, minced), salt and pepper (to taste)
- **Servings:** 4
- **Process:** Mix olive oil, lemon zest, dill, garlic, salt, and pepper. Rub on salmon. Grill for 5-7 mins each side.
- **Shopping List:** Salmon fillets, olive oil, lemon, dill, garlic.
- **Tips:** Let the salmon marinate for 30 mins for enhanced flavor.

Shrimp and Asparagus Stir-Fry

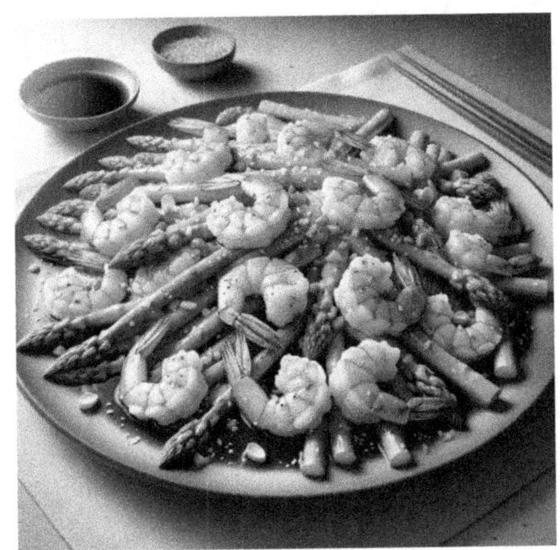

- **P.T.:** 20 mins
- **Ingr.:** Shrimp (1 lb, peeled & deveined), asparagus (1 bunch, trimmed & cut), garlic (2 cloves, minced), soy sauce (low sodium, 2 tbsp), sesame oil (1 tbsp), ginger (1 tsp, grated)
- **Servings:** 4
- **Process:** Stir-fry asparagus and garlic in sesame oil. Add shrimp, ginger, and soy sauce. Cook until shrimp are pink.
- **Shopping List:** Shrimp, asparagus, garlic, low sodium soy sauce, sesame oil, ginger.
- **Tips:** Add a splash of lime juice for a tangy twist.

Baked Cod with Lemon Butter

- **P.T.:** 30 mins
- **Ingr.:** Cod fillets (4), butter (2 tbsp, unsalted), lemon juice (2 tbsp), parsley (1 tbsp, chopped), paprika (1 tsp), salt and pepper (to taste)
- **Servings:** 4
- **Process:** Place cod in baking dish. Mix butter, lemon juice, parsley, and paprika. Pour over cod. Bake at 375°F for 20 mins.
- **Shopping List:** Cod fillets, butter, lemon, parsley, paprika.
- **Tips:** Serve with a side of steamed vegetables for a complete meal.

Scallop and Pea Risotto

- **P.T.:** 45 mins
- **Ingr.:** Scallops (1 lb), Arborio rice (1 cup), vegetable broth (4 cups), peas (1 cup), onion (1, diced), white wine (1/2 cup), Parmesan cheese (1/2 cup, grated), olive oil (1 tbsp)
- **Servings:** 4
- **Process:** Sauté onion in oil, add rice, cook for 1 min. Add wine, then broth gradually. Stir in peas, cook until rice is creamy. Sear scallops, serve on top.
- **Shopping List:** Scallops, Arborio rice, vegetable broth, peas, onion, white wine, Parmesan cheese, olive oil.
- **Tips:** Pat scallops dry before searing for a perfect crust.

Tilapia Tacos with Mango Salsa

- **P.T.:** 30 mins
- **Ingr.:** Tilapia fillets (4), whole wheat tortillas (8), mango (1, diced), red onion (1/4 cup, diced), cilantro (1/4 cup, chopped), lime juice (2 tbsp), chili powder (1 tsp), olive oil (1 tbsp)
- **Servings:** 4
- **Process:** Season tilapia with chili powder, cook in olive oil. Mix mango, onion, cilantro, and lime juice. Serve fish in tortillas, top with salsa.
- **Shopping List:** Tilapia fillets, whole wheat tortillas, mango, red onion, cilantro, lime, chili powder, olive oil.
- **Tips:** Add avocado slices for creaminess.

Mediterranean Baked Trout

- **P.T.:** 35 mins
- **Ingr.:** Trout fillets (4), cherry tomatoes (1 cup, halved), Kalamata olives (1/4 cup, pitted), capers (1 tbsp), lemon slices (8), olive oil (2 tbsp), oregano (1 tsp, dried)
- **Servings:** 4
- **Process:** Place trout on baking sheet, top with tomatoes, olives, capers, lemon, drizzle with oil, sprinkle oregano. Bake at 375°F for 20 mins.
- **Shopping List:** Trout fillets, cherry tomatoes, Kalamata olives, capers, lemon, olive oil, oregano.
- **Tips:** Serve with a side of quinoa or brown rice.

Spicy Garlic Shrimp Zoodles

- **P.T.:** 20 mins
- **Ingr.:** Shrimp (1 lb, peeled & deveined), zucchini (4, spiralized), garlic (3 cloves, minced), red pepper flakes (1/2 tsp), olive oil (2 tbsp), lemon juice (1 tbsp), parsley (1/4 cup, chopped)
- **Servings:** 4
- **Process:** Sauté garlic and red pepper in oil. Add shrimp, cook until pink. Toss with zoodles, lemon juice, parsley.
- **Shopping List:** Shrimp, zucchini, garlic, red pepper flakes, olive oil, lemon, parsley.
- **Tips:** Cook zoodles briefly to retain their crunch.

Chapter 9: Sides to Complement

Vegetable Sides

Roasted Garlic Cauliflower

- **P.T.:** 30 mins
- **Ingr.:** Cauliflower (1 head, cut into florets), olive oil (2 tbsp), garlic (3 cloves, minced), parsley (1 tbsp, chopped), salt and pepper (to taste)
- **Servings:** 4
- **Process:** Toss cauliflower with olive oil, garlic, salt, and pepper. Roast at 400°F for 25 mins. Sprinkle with parsley.
- **Shopping List:** Cauliflower, olive oil, garlic, parsley.
- **Tips:** For extra flavor, add a sprinkle of Parmesan cheese before serving.

Sautéed Green Beans with Almonds

- **P.T.:** 15 mins
- **Ingr.:** Green beans (1 lb, trimmed), slivered almonds (1/4 cup), garlic (2 cloves, minced), olive oil (1 tbsp), lemon juice (1 tbsp), salt and pepper (to taste)
- **Servings:** 4
- **Process:** Sauté green beans and garlic in olive oil. Add almonds, cook until beans are tender. Drizzle with lemon juice.
- **Shopping List:** Green beans, slivered almonds, garlic, olive oil, lemon.
- **Tips:** Blanch green beans beforehand for a quicker cook time.

Balsamic Roasted Brussels Sprouts

- **P.T.:** 35 mins
- **Ingr.:** Brussels sprouts (1 lb, halved), balsamic vinegar (2 tbsp), olive oil (2 tbsp), garlic (1 clove, minced), salt and pepper (to taste)
- **Servings:** 4
- **Process:** Toss Brussels sprouts with oil, vinegar, garlic, salt, and pepper. Roast at 375°F for 30 mins.
- **Shopping List:** Brussels sprouts, balsamic vinegar, olive oil, garlic.
- **Tips:** Roast until edges are crispy and caramelized.

Spicy Roasted Sweet Potatoes

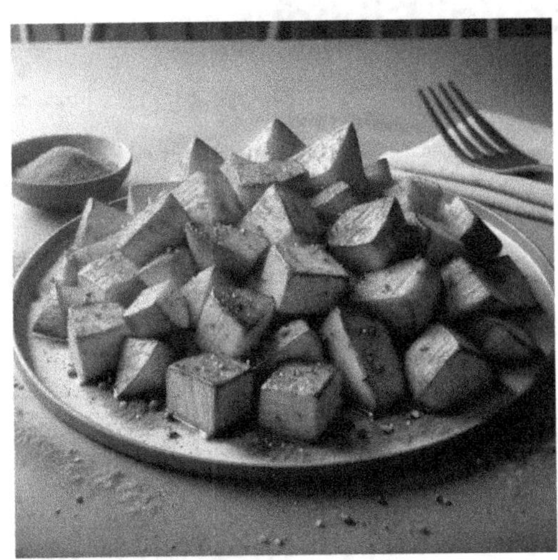

- **P.T.:** 40 mins
- **Ingr.:** Sweet potatoes (2, cubed), olive oil (2 tbsp), paprika (1 tsp), cayenne pepper (1/4 tsp), salt (to taste)
- **Servings:** 4
- **Process:** Toss sweet potatoes with oil, paprika, cayenne, and salt. Bake at 400°F for 35 mins.
- **Shopping List:** Sweet potatoes, olive oil, paprika, cayenne pepper.
- **Tips:** Adjust the amount of cayenne to control the heat level.

Grilled Asparagus with Lemon

- **P.T.:** 15 mins
- **Ingr.:** Asparagus (1 lb, trimmed), olive oil (1 tbsp), lemon (1, zest and juice), salt and pepper (to taste)
- **Servings:** 4
- **Process:** Grill asparagus with olive oil until tender. Drizzle with lemon juice and zest.
- **Shopping List:** Asparagus, olive oil, lemon.
- **Tips:** For a charred flavor, grill asparagus directly over high heat.

Herbed Zucchini Ribbons

- **P.T.:** 10 mins
- **Ingr.:** Zucchini (2, large), olive oil (1 tbsp), mixed herbs (1 tbsp, e.g., basil, thyme), garlic (1 clove, minced), salt and pepper (to taste)
- **Servings:** 4
- **Process:** Use a vegetable peeler to create ribbons from zucchini. Sauté with garlic, herbs, salt, and pepper.
- **Shopping List:** Zucchini, olive oil, mixed herbs, garlic.
- **Tips:** Don't overcook zucchini to maintain its texture.

Stir-Fried Broccoli with Garlic

- **P.T.:** 15 mins
- **Ingr.:** Broccoli (1 head, cut into florets), garlic (3 cloves, minced), olive oil (2 tbsp), soy sauce (1 tbsp, low sodium), sesame seeds (1 tbsp)
- **Servings:** 4
- **Process:** Stir-fry broccoli and garlic in oil. Add soy sauce, cook until broccoli is tender. Sprinkle with sesame seeds.
- **Shopping List:** Broccoli, garlic, olive oil, low sodium soy sauce, sesame seeds.
- **Tips:** Add a splash of water to the pan to help broccoli steam and cook evenly.

Grains and Legumes

Quinoa Tabbouleh

- **P.T.:** 20 mins
- **Ingr.:** Quinoa (1 cup, cooked), cucumber (1, diced), tomatoes (2, diced), parsley (1/2 cup, chopped), mint (1/4 cup, chopped), lemon juice (2 tbsp), olive oil (1 tbsp), salt and pepper (to taste)
- **Servings:** 4
- **Process:** Mix quinoa, cucumber, tomatoes, parsley, and mint. Dress with lemon juice, olive oil, salt, and pepper.
- **Shopping List:** Quinoa, cucumber, tomatoes, parsley, mint, lemon, olive oil.
- **Tips:** Let it sit for an hour for flavors to meld.

Brown Rice and Black Bean Pilaf

- **P.T.:** 45 mins
- **Ingr.:** Brown rice (1 cup), black beans (1 can, drained & rinsed), onion (1, diced), garlic (2 cloves, minced), vegetable broth (2 cups), cumin (1 tsp), olive oil (1 tbsp)
- **Servings:** 4
- **Process:** Sauté onion and garlic in oil. Add rice, beans, cumin, and broth. Simmer until rice is cooked.
- **Shopping List:** Brown rice, black beans, onion, garlic, vegetable broth, cumin, olive oil.
- **Tips:** Add a dash of chili powder for a spicy kick.

Lentil Salad with Mustard Vinaigrette

- **P.T.:** 30 mins
- **Ingr.:** Lentils (1 cup, cooked), cherry tomatoes (1 cup, halved), spinach (1 cup, chopped), red onion (1/4 cup, thinly sliced), Dijon mustard (1 tbsp), apple cider vinegar (2 tbsp), olive oil (2 tbsp), honey (1 tsp, sugar-free)
- **Servings:** 4
- **Process:** Whisk mustard, vinegar, oil, and honey for dressing. Toss lentils, tomatoes, spinach, and onion with dressing.
- **Shopping List:** Lentils, cherry tomatoes, spinach, red onion, Dijon mustard, apple cider vinegar, olive oil, sugar-free honey.
- **Tips:** Serve chilled or at room temperature.

Barley and Roasted Vegetable Medley

- **P.T.:** 55 mins
- **Ingr.:** Barley (1 cup), assorted vegetables (e.g., bell peppers, zucchini, carrots, 2 cups chopped), olive oil (2 tbsp), thyme (1 tsp), vegetable broth (2 cups)
- **Servings:** 4
- **Process:** Roast vegetables with olive oil and thyme at 400°F for 25 mins. Cook barley in broth. Combine barley and vegetables.
- **Shopping List:** Barley, bell peppers, zucchini, carrots, olive oil, thyme, vegetable broth.
- **Tips:** Add a squeeze of lemon for a fresh flavor.

Couscous with Sun-Dried Tomatoes and Olives

- **P.T.:** 20 mins
- **Ingr.:** Couscous (1 cup), sun-dried tomatoes (1/2 cup, chopped), Kalamata olives (1/4 cup, pitted & chopped), parsley (1/4 cup, chopped), lemon juice (2 tbsp), olive oil (1 tbsp)
- **Servings:** 4
- **Process:** Prepare couscous as per package instructions. Mix in tomatoes, olives, parsley, lemon juice, and olive oil.
- **Shopping List:** Couscous, sun-dried tomatoes, Kalamata olives, parsley, lemon, olive oil.
- **Tips:** Fluff couscous with a fork after cooking for the best texture.

Garlic and Herb Bulgar Wheat

- **P.T.:** 25 mins
- **Ingr.:** Bulgar wheat (1 cup), garlic (2 cloves, minced), mixed herbs (e.g., rosemary, thyme, 1 tbsp, chopped), vegetable broth (2 cups), olive oil (1 tbsp)
- **Servings:** 4
- **Process:** Sauté garlic and herbs in oil. Add bulgar wheat, cook for 1 min. Add broth, simmer until absorbed.
- **Shopping List:** Bulgar wheat, garlic, mixed herbs, vegetable broth, olive oil.
- **Tips:** Perfect as a side for grilled meats or vegetables.

Millet Pilaf with Vegetables

- **P.T.:** 30 mins
- **Ingr.:** Millet (1 cup), mixed vegetables (e.g., peas, carrots, 2 cups), onion (1, diced), vegetable broth (2 1/2 cups), olive oil (1 tbsp), parsley (1 tbsp, chopped)
- **Servings:** 4
- **Process:** Sauté onion in oil. Add millet, toast for 2 mins. Add vegetables, broth. Simmer until millet is cooked and fluffy.
- **Shopping List:** Millet, peas, carrots, onion, vegetable broth, olive oil, parsley.
- **Tips:** Toasting millet before cooking enhances its nutty flavor.

Creative Carb Alternatives

Cauliflower Rice Pilaf

- **P.T.:** 20 mins
- **Ingr.:** Cauliflower (1 head, riced), onion (1, diced), garlic (2 cloves, minced), carrots (1/2 cup, diced), peas (1/2 cup), olive oil (2 tbsp), cumin (1 tsp), salt and pepper (to taste)
- **Servings:** 4
- **Process:** Sauté onion and garlic in olive oil. Add cauliflower rice, carrots, peas, and cumin. Cook until tender.
- **Shopping List:** Cauliflower, onion, garlic, carrots, peas, olive oil, cumin.
- **Tips:** Use a food processor to rice the cauliflower quickly.

Zucchini Noodles (Zoodles) with Pesto

- **P.T.:** 15 mins
- **Ingr.:** Zucchini (4, spiralized), basil pesto (1/4 cup), cherry tomatoes (1 cup, halved), Parmesan cheese (for garnish), olive oil (1 tbsp)
- **Servings:** 4
- **Process:** Sauté zoodles in olive oil for 2-3 mins. Toss with pesto and tomatoes. Garnish with Parmesan.
- **Shopping List:** Zucchini, basil pesto, cherry tomatoes, Parmesan cheese, olive oil.
- **Tips:** Don't overcook the zoodles to maintain their texture.

Spaghetti Squash with Garlic and Herbs

- **P.T.:** 1 hr
- **Ingr.:** Spaghetti squash (1, halved and seeded), garlic (3 cloves, minced), parsley (1/4 cup, chopped), olive oil (2 tbsp), salt and pepper (to taste)
- **Servings:** 4
- **Process:** Roast squash at 400°F for 40 mins. Scrape into strands. Sauté garlic in oil, toss with squash, parsley, salt, and pepper.
- **Shopping List:** Spaghetti squash, garlic, parsley, olive oil.
- **Tips:** Mix in some chili flakes for a spicy version.

Butternut Squash Mash

- **P.T.:** 35 mins
- **Ingr.:** Butternut squash (1, peeled & cubed), butter (2 tbsp, unsalted), cinnamon (1/2 tsp), nutmeg (a pinch), salt and pepper (to taste)
- **Servings:** 4
- **Process:** Boil squash until tender. Mash with butter, cinnamon, nutmeg, salt, and pepper.
- **Shopping List:** Butternut squash, butter, cinnamon, nutmeg.
- **Tips:** Add a splash of almond milk for creaminess.

Baked Eggplant Fries

- **P.T.:** 30 mins
- **Ingr.:** Eggplant (1, sliced into fries), almond flour (1/2 cup), Parmesan cheese (1/4 cup, grated), garlic powder (1 tsp), olive oil (for brushing), salt and pepper (to taste)
- **Servings:** 4
- **Process:** Coat eggplant in almond flour, Parmesan, garlic powder, salt, and pepper. Brush with oil. Bake at 425°F for 20 mins.
- **Shopping List:** Eggplant, almond flour, Parmesan cheese, garlic powder, olive oil.
- **Tips:** Serve with a yogurt-based dipping sauce.

Roasted Turnip Wedges

- **P.T.:** 40 mins
- **Ingr.:** Turnips (3, cut into wedges), olive oil (2 tbsp), rosemary (1 tsp, chopped), garlic powder (1/2 tsp), salt and pepper (to taste)
- **Servings:** 4
- **Process:** Toss turnips with oil, rosemary, garlic powder, salt, and pepper. Roast at 400°F for 30 mins.
- **Shopping List:** Turnips, olive oil, rosemary, garlic powder.
- **Tips:** Turnips can be parboiled before roasting for a softer texture.

- **P.T.:** 20 mins
- **Ingr.:** Kale (1 bunch, torn into pieces), olive oil (1 tbsp), Parmesan cheese (2 tbsp, grated), salt (to taste)
- **Servings:** 4
- **Process:** Toss kale with olive oil and salt. Bake at 300°F for 15 mins. Sprinkle with Parmesan.
- **Shopping List:** Kale, olive oil, Parmesan cheese.
- **Tips:** Ensure kale is dry before baking for crispier chips.

Chapter 10: Guilt-Free Desserts

Fruit-Based Desserts

Baked Cinnamon Apples

- **P.T.:** 30 mins
- **Ingr.:** Apples (4, cored and sliced), cinnamon (1 tsp), nutmeg (1/4 tsp), stevia (2 tbsp), water (1/4 cup)
- **Servings:** 4
- **Process:** Toss apple slices with cinnamon, nutmeg, and stevia. Place in a baking dish, add water. Bake at 350°F for 25 mins.
- **Shopping List:** Apples, cinnamon, nutmeg, stevia.
- **Tips:** Serve with sugar-free vanilla yogurt for added creaminess.

Berry Salad with Lemon Drizzle

- **P.T.:** 15 mins
- **Ingr.:** Mixed berries (2 cups), lemon juice (2 tbsp), lemon zest (1 tsp), stevia (1 tbsp), mint leaves (for garnish)
- **Servings:** 4
- **Process:** Combine berries, lemon juice, zest, and stevia. Chill before serving. Garnish with mint.
- **Shopping List:** Mixed berries, lemon, stevia, mint leaves.
- **Tips:** Use fresh, seasonal berries for the best flavor.

Grilled Peaches with Cinnamon

- **P.T.:** 20 mins
- **Ingr.:** Peaches (4, halved and pitted), cinnamon (1 tsp), butter (2 tbsp, unsalted), stevia (1 tbsp)
- **Servings:** 4
- **Process:** Brush peaches with butter and sprinkle with cinnamon and stevia. Grill on medium heat for 4-5 mins per side.
- **Shopping List:** Peaches, cinnamon, butter, stevia.
- **Tips:** Serve with a dollop of Greek yogurt.

Pineapple and Mango Salsa

- **P.T.:** 15 mins
- **Ingr.:** Pineapple (1 cup, diced), mango (1 cup, diced), red bell pepper (1/4 cup, diced), red onion (2 tbsp, minced), cilantro (2 tbsp, chopped), lime juice (2 tbsp), jalapeño (1, minced, optional)
- **Servings:** 4
- **Process:** Combine all ingredients. Let sit for 10 mins before serving.
- **Shopping List:** Pineapple, mango, red bell pepper, red onion, cilantro, lime, jalapeño.
- **Tips:** Adjust jalapeño quantity for desired spiciness.

Kiwi and Berry Parfait

- **P.T.:** 10 mins
- **Ingr.:** Kiwi (2, peeled and sliced), mixed berries (1 cup), Greek yogurt (1 cup, sugar-free), granola (1/2 cup, sugar-free), honey (1 tbsp, sugar-free)
- **Servings:** 2
- **Process:** Layer yogurt, granola, kiwi, and berries in glasses. Drizzle with honey.
- **Shopping List:** Kiwi, mixed berries, Greek yogurt, granola, sugar-free honey.
- **Tips:** Layer the parfait just before serving to keep granola crunchy.

Baked Pears with Walnuts

- **P.T.:** 35 mins
- **Ingr.:** Pears (4, halved and cored), walnuts (1/4 cup, chopped), cinnamon (1 tsp), stevia (2 tbsp), butter (2 tbsp)
- **Servings:** 4
- **Process:** Place pears on a baking sheet. Mix walnuts, cinnamon, and stevia. Fill pear halves, top with a dot of butter. Bake at 350°F for 30 mins.
- **Shopping List:** Pears, walnuts, cinnamon, stevia, butter.
- **Tips:** Serve warm with a scoop of sugar-free ice cream.

Watermelon and Feta Salad

- **P.T.:** 15 mins
- **Ingr.:** Watermelon (4 cups, cubed), feta cheese (1/2 cup, crumbled), mint leaves (1/4 cup, chopped), balsamic glaze (2 tbsp), olive oil (1 tbsp), black pepper (to taste)
- **Servings:** 4
- **Process:** Toss watermelon with feta and mint. Drizzle with balsamic glaze and olive oil. Sprinkle with black pepper.
- **Shopping List:** Watermelon, feta cheese, mint leaves, balsamic glaze, olive oil.
- **Tips:** Chill the watermelon before preparing for a refreshing treat.

Sugar-Free Treats

Almond Flour Chocolate Chip Cookies

- **P.T.:** 25 mins
- **Ingr.:** Almond flour (2 cups), erythritol (1 cup, granulated), unsalted butter (1/2 cup, softened), egg (1), vanilla extract (1 tsp), sugar-free chocolate chips (1/2 cup), baking soda (1 tsp), salt (a pinch)
- **Servings:** 12 cookies
- **Process:** Cream butter and erythritol. Add egg, vanilla. Mix in almond flour, baking soda, salt. Fold in chocolate chips. Drop spoonfuls on a baking sheet. Bake at 350°F for 12-15 mins.
- **Shopping List:** Almond flour, erythritol, butter, egg, vanilla extract, sugar-free chocolate chips, baking soda.
- **Tips:** Let cookies cool on the baking sheet for firmness.

No-Bake Peanut Butter Balls

- **P.T.:** 15 mins (plus chilling)
- **Ingr.:** Peanut butter (1 cup, unsweetened), coconut flour (1/2 cup), stevia (1/4 cup), dark chocolate (1/2 cup, sugar-free, melted), vanilla extract (1 tsp)
- **Servings:** 15 balls
- **Process:** Mix peanut butter, coconut flour, stevia, and vanilla. Roll into balls. Dip in melted chocolate. Chill until set.
- **Shopping List:** Peanut butter, coconut flour, stevia, sugar-free dark chocolate, vanilla extract.
- **Tips:** Store in the refrigerator for up to a week.

Sugar-Free Lemon Bars

- **P.T.:** 40 mins
- **Ingr.:** Almond flour (for crust, 1 1/2 cups), butter (for crust, 1/4 cup, melted), erythritol (1 cup, for filling), eggs (3, for filling), lemon juice (1/2 cup), lemon zest (1 tbsp)
- **Servings:** 9 bars
- **Process:** Mix almond flour and butter, press into a pan. Bake at 350°F for 10 mins. Whisk eggs, erythritol, lemon juice, zest. Pour over crust, bake for 20 mins.
- **Shopping List:** Almond flour, butter, erythritol, eggs, lemons.
- **Tips:** Cool completely before cutting into bars.

Avocado Chocolate Mousse

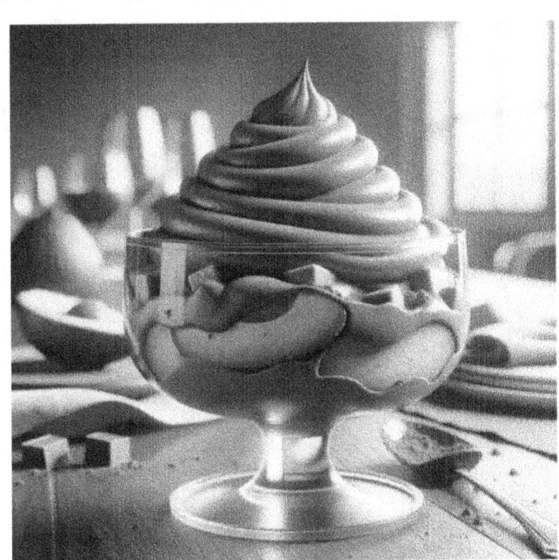

- **P.T.:** 10 mins
- **Ingr.:** Ripe avocados (2), cocoa powder (1/4 cup), erythritol (1/4 cup), almond milk (1/4 cup), vanilla extract (1 tsp)
- **Servings:** 4
- **Process:** Blend avocados, cocoa powder, erythritol, almond milk, vanilla until smooth.
- **Shopping List:** Avocados, cocoa powder, erythritol, almond milk, vanilla extract.
- **Tips:** Chill for an hour before serving for a firmer texture.

Coconut Flour Pancakes

- **P.T.:** 20 mins
- **Ingr.:** Coconut flour (1/2 cup), eggs (4), almond milk (1/2 cup), stevia (2 tbsp), baking powder (1 tsp), vanilla extract (1 tsp)
- **Servings:** 6 pancakes
- **Process:** Whisk eggs, almond milk, stevia, vanilla. Add coconut flour, baking powder. Cook on a griddle over medium heat.
- **Shopping List:** Coconut flour, eggs, almond milk, stevia, baking powder, vanilla extract.
- **Tips:** Serve with sugar-free syrup or fresh berries.

Baked Raspberry Ripple Cheesecake

- **P.T.:** 1 hr 10 mins
- **Ingr.:** Cream cheese (2 cups), eggs (3), erythritol (3/4 cup), vanilla extract (1 tsp), raspberries (1 cup), almond flour (for crust, 1 cup), butter (for crust, 1/4 cup)
- **Servings:** 8 slices
- **Process:** Mix almond flour and butter, press into a pan. Blend cream cheese, eggs, erythritol, vanilla. Pour over crust. Swirl in raspberries. Bake at 325°F for 50 mins.
- **Shopping List:** Cream cheese, eggs, erythritol, vanilla extract, raspberries, almond flour, butter.
- **Tips:** Let cheesecake cool in the oven gradually to prevent cracks.

Dark Chocolate Almond Bark

- **P.T.:** 30 mins (plus chilling)
- **Ingr.:** Dark chocolate (70% or higher, sugar-free, 1 cup), almonds (1/2 cup, toasted and chopped), sea salt (a pinch)
- **Servings:** 8 pieces
- **Process:** Melt chocolate, stir in half the almonds. Spread on a lined tray. Top with remaining almonds, salt. Chill until set.
- **Shopping List:** Sugar-free dark chocolate, almonds, sea salt.
- **Tips:** Break into rustic pieces for serving.

Baked Goodies

Almond and Blueberry Muffins

- **P.T.:** 35 mins
- **Ingr.:** Almond flour (2 cups), eggs (3), unsweetened applesauce (1/2 cup), erythritol (1/2 cup), baking powder (1 tsp), vanilla extract (1 tsp), blueberries (1 cup)
- **Servings:** 12 muffins
- **Process:** Mix almond flour, erythritol, and baking powder. Add eggs, applesauce, vanilla. Fold in blueberries. Bake in muffin tins at 350°F for 25 mins.
- **Shopping List:** Almond flour, eggs, unsweetened applesauce, erythritol, vanilla extract, blueberries.
- **Tips:** Use fresh or frozen blueberries.

Carrot and Walnut Cake

- **P.T.:** 50 mins
- **Ingr.:** Grated carrots (2 cups), eggs (4), almond flour (1 1/2 cups), erythritol (3/4 cup), cinnamon (1 tsp), nutmeg (1/2 tsp), walnuts (1/2 cup, chopped), baking powder (1 tsp)
- **Servings:** 8 slices
- **Process:** Whisk eggs, erythritol. Add almond flour, baking powder, spices. Stir in carrots, walnuts. Bake at 350°F for 35 mins.
- **Shopping List:** Carrots, eggs, almond flour, erythritol, cinnamon, nutmeg, walnuts.
- **Tips:** Cool completely before slicing.

Sugar-Free Banana Bread

- **P.T.:** 1 hr
- **Ingr.:** Ripe bananas (3), eggs (3), almond flour (2 cups), erythritol (1/2 cup), baking soda (1 tsp), vanilla extract (1 tsp)
- **Servings:** 10 slices
- **Process:** Mash bananas. Mix with beaten eggs, erythritol, vanilla. Add almond flour, baking soda. Pour into loaf pan, bake at 350°F for 50 mins.
- **Shopping List:** Bananas, eggs, almond flour, erythritol, vanilla extract.
- **Tips:** Add nuts or dark chocolate chips for variation.

Pumpkin Spice Cookies

- **P.T.:** 30 mins
- **Ingr.:** Pumpkin puree (1 cup), almond flour (2 cups), erythritol (1/2 cup), eggs (2), pumpkin pie spice (1 tbsp), baking powder (1 tsp)
- **Servings:** 15 cookies
- **Process:** Mix pumpkin, eggs, erythritol. Add almond flour, spice, baking powder. Drop spoonfuls on baking sheet, bake at 350°F for 20 mins.
- **Shopping List:** Pumpkin puree, almond flour, erythritol, eggs, pumpkin pie spice.
- **Tips:** Press cookies down before baking for even cooking.

Chocolate Zucchini Bread

- **P.T.:** 1 hr
- **Ingr.:** Grated zucchini (1 1/2 cups), almond flour (1 3/4 cups), cocoa powder (1/4 cup), eggs (3), erythritol (3/4 cup), vanilla extract (1 tsp), baking soda (1 tsp)
- **Servings:** 10 slices
- **Process:** Mix zucchini, eggs, erythritol, vanilla. Add almond flour, cocoa, baking soda. Bake in loaf pan at 350°F for 45 mins.
- **Shopping List:** Zucchini, almond flour, cocoa powder, eggs, erythritol, vanilla extract.
- **Tips:** Squeeze excess moisture from zucchini.

Lemon Poppy Seed Loaf

- **P.T.:** 55 mins
- **Ingr.:** Almond flour (2 cups), eggs (4), erythritol (1/2 cup), lemon juice (1/4 cup), lemon zest (1 tbsp), poppy seeds (2 tbsp), baking powder (1 tsp)
- **Servings:** 8 slices
- **Process:** Whisk eggs, erythritol, lemon juice, zest. Add almond flour, baking powder, poppy seeds. Bake at 350°F in loaf pan for 40 mins.
- **Shopping List:** Almond flour, eggs, erythritol, lemons, poppy seeds.
- **Tips:** Glaze with a sugar-free lemon drizzle.

Apple Cinnamon Scones

- **P.T.:** 30 mins
- **Ingr.:** Almond flour (2 cups), diced apples (1 cup), eggs (2), erythritol (1/4 cup), cinnamon (1 tsp), baking powder (1 tsp), butter (1/4 cup, cold and cubed)
- **Servings:** 8 scones
- **Process:** Mix almond flour, erythritol, cinnamon, baking powder. Add butter, eggs. Fold in apples. Form scones, bake at 375°F for 20 mins.
- **Shopping List:** Almond flour, apples, eggs, erythritol, cinnamon, butter.
- **Tips:** Serve with a pat of butter or sugar-free jam.

Chapter 11: Drinks and Smoothies

Refreshing Beverages

Cucumber Mint Infused Water

- **P.T.:** 5 mins (plus chilling time)
- **Ingr.:** Cucumber (1, thinly sliced), fresh mint leaves (10), water (1 liter)
- **Servings:** 4
- **Process:** Combine cucumber slices, mint leaves, and water in a pitcher. Refrigerate for at least 1 hour before serving.
- **Shopping List:** Cucumber, fresh mint, water.
- **Tips:** Add a few slices of lemon for an extra zing.

Ginger Turmeric Tea

- **P.T.:** 15 mins
- **Ingr.:** Fresh ginger root (2 inches, sliced), turmeric powder (1 tsp), lemon juice (2 tbsp), honey (sugar-free, 1 tbsp), water (4 cups)
- **Servings:** 4
- **Process:** Boil ginger in water for 10 mins. Add turmeric, simmer for 5 more mins. Strain, add lemon juice and honey.
- **Shopping List:** Fresh ginger root, turmeric powder, lemon, sugar-free honey, water.
- **Tips:** Adjust the amount of ginger for desired spiciness.

Berry Lemonade

- **P.T.:** 10 mins
- **Ingr.:** Mixed berries (1 cup), lemon juice (1/2 cup), stevia (to taste), water (3 cups)
- **Servings:** 4
- **Process:** Blend berries with lemon juice and water. Strain, sweeten with stevia.
- **Shopping List:** Mixed berries, lemons, stevia, water.
- **Tips:** Use a mix of berries like strawberries, raspberries, and blueberries for a rich flavor.

Nutritious Smoothies

Spinach and Avocado Smoothie

- **P.T.:** 10 mins
- **Ingr.:** Spinach (2 cups), avocado (1/2, ripe), Greek yogurt (1/2 cup, unsweetened), almond milk (1 cup), stevia (to taste), ice cubes (1/2 cup)
- **Servings:** 2
- **Process:** Blend all ingredients until smooth.
- **Shopping List:** Spinach, avocado, Greek yogurt, almond milk, stevia, ice cubes.
- **Tips:** Add a scoop of protein powder for an extra boost.

Blueberry and Flaxseed Smoothie

- **P.T.:** 10 mins
- **Ingr.:** Blueberries (1 cup, frozen), flaxseed (2 tbsp, ground), Greek yogurt (1/2 cup, unsweetened), almond milk (1 cup), cinnamon (1/2 tsp)
- **Servings:** 2
- **Process:** Blend all ingredients until smooth.
- **Shopping List:** Blueberries, ground flaxseed, Greek yogurt, almond milk, cinnamon.
- **Tips:** Add a few drops of vanilla extract for extra flavor.

Kale and Berry Smoothie

- **P.T.:** 10 mins
- **Ingr.:** Kale (1 cup, chopped), mixed berries (1 cup, frozen), banana (1), almond milk (1 cup), chia seeds (1 tbsp)
- **Servings:** 2
- **Process:** Blend all ingredients until smooth.
- **Shopping List:** Kale, mixed berries, banana, almond milk, chia seeds.
- **Tips:** Freeze the banana beforehand for a creamier texture.

Herbal Teas and Infusions

Chamomile and Lavender Tea

- **P.T.:** 10 mins
- **Ingr.:** Chamomile flowers (1 tbsp), lavender buds (1 tsp), boiling water (2 cups)
- **Servings:** 2
- **Process:** Steep chamomile and lavender in boiling water for 8 mins. Strain and serve.
- **Shopping List:** Chamomile flowers, lavender buds.
- **Tips:** Add a slice of lemon or a dollop of honey for added flavor.

Peppermint and Lemon Balm Tea

- **P.T.:** 10 mins
- **Ingr.:** Fresh peppermint leaves (1/4 cup), lemon balm leaves (1/4 cup), boiling water (2 cups)
- **Servings:** 2
- **Process:** Steep peppermint and lemon balm in boiling water for 7 mins. Strain and serve.
- **Shopping List:** Fresh peppermint leaves, lemon balm leaves.
- **Tips:** Enjoy this tea after meals to aid digestion.

Ginger and Turmeric Infusion

- **P.T.:** 15 mins
- **Ingr.:** Fresh ginger (2 inches, sliced), turmeric root (1 inch, sliced), lemon juice (2 tbsp), boiling water (2 cups)
- **Servings:** 2
- **Process:** Simmer ginger and turmeric in boiling water for 10 mins. Add lemon juice, strain, and serve.
- **Shopping List:** Fresh ginger, turmeric root, lemon.
- **Tips:** Sweeten with a teaspoon of sugar-free honey if desired.

Chapter 12: 45-Day Meal Plan for Type 2 Diabetes

0-10 Meal Plan:

Day	Breakfast	Snack 1	Lunch	Snack 2	Dinner	Side
1	Egg-Veggie Scramble	Zucchini and Carrot Ribbon Salad	Spinach and Avocado Delight	Greek Yogurt and Berry Cups	Chickpea and Spinach Curry	Sautéed Green Beans with Almonds
2	Berry Yogurt Parfait	Cucumber Hummus Bites	Arugula and Pear Salad	Avocado and Tomato Salad	Zucchini Lasagna Rolls	Balsamic Roasted Brussels Sprouts
3	Avocado Toast Delight	Almond-Stuffed Dates	Minty Watermelon and Feta Salad	Kale Chips with Nutritional Yeast	Stuffed Bell Peppers with Quinoa	Spicy Roasted Sweet Potatoes
4	Smoothie Sunrise	Greek Yogurt and Berry Cups	Classic Caesar with a Twist	Spiced Roasted Chickpeas	Vegetable Stir-Fry with Tofu	Grilled Asparagus with Lemon
5	Cottage Cheese and Pineapple Bowl	Avocado and Tomato Salad	Mixed Greens with Raspberry Vinaigrette	Zucchini and Carrot Ribbon Salad	Portobello Mushroom Fajitas	Herbed Zucchini Ribbons
6	Power Seed Pudding	Kale Chips with Nutritional Yeast	Beet and Goat Cheese Salad	Cucumber Hummus Bites	Lentil Sloppy Joes	Stir-Fried Broccoli with Garlic
7	Morning Zest Oat Bowl	Spiced Roasted Chickpeas	Kale and Quinoa Power Salad	Almond-Stuffed Dates	Eggplant Parmesan Stack	Roasted Garlic Cauliflower
8	Egg-Veggie Scramble	Zucchini and Carrot Ribbon Salad	Spinach and Avocado Delight	Greek Yogurt and Berry Cups	Chickpea and Spinach Curry	Sautéed Green Beans with Almonds
9	Berry Yogurt Parfait	Cucumber Hummus Bites	Arugula and Pear Salad	Avocado and Tomato Salad	Zucchini Lasagna Rolls	Balsamic Roasted Brussels Sprouts
10	Avocado Toast Delight	Almond-Stuffed Dates	Minty Watermelon and Feta Salad	Kale Chips with Nutritional Yeast	Stuffed Bell Peppers with Quinoa	Spicy Roasted Sweet Potatoes

11-20 Meal Plan:

Day	Breakfast	Snack 1	Lunch	Snack 2	Dinner	Side
11	Smoothie Sunrise	Greek Yogurt and Berry Cups	Classic Caesar with a Twist	Spiced Roasted Chickpeas	Vegetable Stir-Fry with Tofu	Grilled Asparagus with Lemon
12	Cottage Cheese and Pineapple Bowl	Avocado and Tomato Salad	Mixed Greens with Raspberry Vinaigrette	Zucchini and Carrot Ribbon Salad	Portobello Mushroom Fajitas	Herbed Zucchini Ribbons
13	Power Seed Pudding	Kale Chips with Nutritional Yeast	Beet and Goat Cheese Salad	Cucumber Hummus Bites	Lentil Sloppy Joes	Stir-Fried Broccoli with Garlic
14	Morning Zest Oat Bowl	Spiced Roasted Chickpeas	Kale and Quinoa Power Salad	Almond-Stuffed Dates	Eggplant Parmesan Stack	Roasted Garlic Cauliflower
15	Egg-Veggie Scramble	Zucchini and Carrot Ribbon Salad	Spinach and Avocado Delight	Greek Yogurt and Berry Cups	Chickpea and Spinach Curry	Sautéed Green Beans with Almonds
16	Berry Yogurt Parfait	Cucumber Hummus Bites	Arugula and Pear Salad	Avocado and Tomato Salad	Zucchini Lasagna Rolls	Balsamic Roasted Brussels Sprouts
17	Avocado Toast Delight	Almond-Stuffed Dates	Minty Watermelon and Feta Salad	Kale Chips with Nutritional Yeast	Stuffed Bell Peppers with Quinoa	Spicy Roasted Sweet Potatoes
18	Smoothie Sunrise	Greek Yogurt and Berry Cups	Classic Caesar with a Twist	Spiced Roasted Chickpeas	Vegetable Stir-Fry with Tofu	Grilled Asparagus with Lemon
19	Cottage Cheese and Pineapple Bowl	Avocado and Tomato Salad	Mixed Greens with Raspberry Vinaigrette	Zucchini and Carrot Ribbon Salad	Portobello Mushroom Fajitas	Herbed Zucchini Ribbons
20	Power Seed Pudding	Kale Chips with Nutritional Yeast	Beet and Goat Cheese Salad	Cucumber Hummus Bites	Lentil Sloppy Joes	Stir-Fried Broccoli with Garlic

21-30 Meal Plan:

Day	Breakfast	Snack 1	Lunch	Snack 2	Dinner	Side
21	Morning Zest Oat Bowl	Spiced Roasted Chickpeas	Kale and Quinoa Power Salad	Almond-Stuffed Dates	Eggplant Parmesan Stack	Roasted Garlic Cauliflower
22	Egg-Veggie Scramble	Zucchini and Carrot Ribbon Salad	Spinach and Avocado Delight	Greek Yogurt and Berry Cups	Chickpea and Spinach Curry	Sautéed Green Beans with Almonds
23	Berry Yogurt Parfait	Cucumber Hummus Bites	Arugula and Pear Salad	Avocado and Tomato Salad	Zucchini Lasagna Rolls	Balsamic Roasted Brussels Sprouts
24	Avocado Toast Delight	Almond-Stuffed Dates	Minty Watermelon and Feta Salad	Kale Chips with Nutritional Yeast	Stuffed Bell Peppers with Quinoa	Spicy Roasted Sweet Potatoes
25	Smoothie Sunrise	Greek Yogurt and Berry Cups	Classic Caesar with a Twist	Spiced Roasted Chickpeas	Vegetable Stir-Fry with Tofu	Grilled Asparagus with Lemon
26	Cottage Cheese and Pineapple Bowl	Avocado and Tomato Salad	Mixed Greens with Raspberry Vinaigrette	Zucchini and Carrot Ribbon Salad	Portobello Mushroom Fajitas	Herbed Zucchini Ribbons
27	Power Seed Pudding	Kale Chips with Nutritional Yeast	Beet and Goat Cheese Salad	Cucumber Hummus Bites	Lentil Sloppy Joes	Stir-Fried Broccoli with Garlic
28	Morning Zest Oat Bowl	Spiced Roasted Chickpeas	Kale and Quinoa Power Salad	Almond-Stuffed Dates	Eggplant Parmesan Stack	Roasted Garlic Cauliflower
29	Egg-Veggie Scramble	Zucchini and Carrot Ribbon Salad	Spinach and Avocado Delight	Greek Yogurt and Berry Cups	Chickpea and Spinach Curry	Sautéed Green Beans with Almonds
30	Berry Yogurt Parfait	Cucumber Hummus Bites	Arugula and Pear Salad	Avocado and Tomato Salad	Zucchini Lasagna Rolls	Balsamic Roasted Brussels Sprouts

31-40 Meal Plan:

Day	Breakfast	Snack 1	Lunch	Snack 2	Dinner	Side
31	Avocado Toast Delight	Almond-Stuffed Dates	Minty Watermelon and Feta Salad	Kale Chips with Nutritional Yeast	Stuffed Bell Peppers with Quinoa	Spicy Roasted Sweet Potatoes
32	Smoothie Sunrise	Greek Yogurt and Berry Cups	Classic Caesar with a Twist	Spiced Roasted Chickpeas	Vegetable Stir-Fry with Tofu	Grilled Asparagus with Lemon
33	Cottage Cheese and Pineapple Bowl	Avocado and Tomato Salad	Mixed Greens with Raspberry Vinaigrette	Zucchini and Carrot Ribbon Salad	Portobello Mushroom Fajitas	Herbed Zucchini Ribbons
34	Power Seed Pudding	Kale Chips with Nutritional Yeast	Beet and Goat Cheese Salad	Cucumber Hummus Bites	Lentil Sloppy Joes	Stir-Fried Broccoli with Garlic
35	Morning Zest Oat Bowl	Spiced Roasted Chickpeas	Kale and Quinoa Power Salad	Almond-Stuffed Dates	Eggplant Parmesan Stack	Roasted Garlic Cauliflower
36	Egg-Veggie Scramble	Zucchini and Carrot Ribbon Salad	Spinach and Avocado Delight	Greek Yogurt and Berry Cups	Chickpea and Spinach Curry	Sautéed Green Beans with Almonds
37	Berry Yogurt Parfait	Cucumber Hummus Bites	Arugula and Pear Salad	Avocado and Tomato Salad	Zucchini Lasagna Rolls	Balsamic Roasted Brussels Sprouts
38	Avocado Toast Delight	Almond-Stuffed Dates	Minty Watermelon and Feta Salad	Kale Chips with Nutritional Yeast	Stuffed Bell Peppers with Quinoa	Spicy Roasted Sweet Potatoes
39	Smoothie Sunrise	Greek Yogurt and Berry Cups	Classic Caesar with a Twist	Spiced Roasted Chickpeas	Vegetable Stir-Fry with Tofu	Grilled Asparagus with Lemon
40	Cottage Cheese and Pineapple Bowl	Avocado and Tomato Salad	Mixed Greens with Raspberry Vinaigrette	Zucchini and Carrot Ribbon Salad	Portobello Mushroom Fajitas	Herbed Zucchini Ribbons

41-45 Meal Plan:

Day	Breakfast	Snack 1	Lunch	Snack 2	Dinner	Side
41	Power Seed Pudding	Kale Chips with Nutritional Yeast	Beet and Goat Cheese Salad	Cucumber Hummus Bites	Lentil Sloppy Joes	Stir-Fried Broccoli with Garlic
42	Morning Zest Oat Bowl	Spiced Roasted Chickpeas	Kale and Quinoa Power Salad	Almond-Stuffed Dates	Eggplant Parmesan Stack	Roasted Garlic Cauliflower
43	Egg-Veggie Scramble	Zucchini and Carrot Ribbon Salad	Spinach and Avocado Delight	Greek Yogurt and Berry Cups	Chickpea and Spinach Curry	Sautéed Green Beans with Almonds
44	Berry Yogurt Parfait	Cucumber Hummus Bites	Arugula and Pear Salad	Avocado and Tomato Salad	Zucchini Lasagna Rolls	Balsamic Roasted Brussels Sprouts
45	Avocado Toast Delight	Almond-Stuffed Dates	Minty Watermelon and Feta Salad	Kale Chips with Nutritional Yeast	Stuffed Bell Peppers with Quinoa	Spicy Roasted Sweet Potatoes

Chapter 13: Moving Forward: A Sustainable Approach

Building Healthy Habits

Embarking on a journey toward better health, especially when managing Type 2 Diabetes, is akin to navigating a river with its ebbs and flows. The key to this journey is building healthy habits that not only align with your diabetes management but also integrate seamlessly into the tapestry of your daily life. It's about creating a sustainable balance that resonates with your personal routine, preferences, and goals.

Imagine, for a moment, the gentle yet persistent growth of a garden. Just as a gardener cultivates the soil, plants the seeds, and nurtures them with consistent care, so too must we tend to the seeds of our new habits. These habits, from mindful eating to regular physical activity, don't sprout overnight. They require nurturing—time, patience, and a gentle yet persistent approach.

Consider the act of mindful eating, a practice not just of choosing foods that are conducive to managing blood sugar levels but also of being present during meals. It's about savoring flavors, acknowledging textures, and honoring the experience of nourishment. This practice extends beyond the table, encompassing the choices made while shopping for groceries or planning meals, encouraging a deeper connection with the food journey from source to plate.

Incorporating physical activity into daily life is another cornerstone of this journey. It need not be an overwhelming venture; small, consistent steps make a vast difference. A brisk morning walk, a cycle through the neighborhood park, or even stretching exercises during a TV show commercial break—these are droplets that create ripples, leading to waves of change in physical well-being.

Moreover, regular monitoring of blood sugar levels, coupled with an awareness of how different foods and activities influence these levels, is paramount. This self-awareness fosters a deeper understanding of your body's responses, guiding you toward choices that maintain a harmonious balance in your health.

As you embark on this journey, remember that building healthy habits is a process of learning, adapting, and growing. It's not about perfection but progress. Each day offers a new canvas to paint with choices that nurture your well-being, and each decision is a brushstroke that contributes to the masterpiece of your health journey.

Staying Motivated

One of the most effective ways to sustain motivation is to celebrate the milestones, no matter how small they may seem. Did you choose a salad over a slice of pizza? That's a victory. Managed a 15-minute walk? Another triumph. These accomplishments, when acknowledged, act like stars in the night sky, guiding and encouraging you to press on.

It's also imperative to remember that motivation is not a constant companion. There will be days when it wanes, shadowed by the challenges of managing a chronic condition. During such times, lean on your support system—family, friends, or a community of fellow journeyers. Sharing your struggles, victories, and insights can reignite the spark of motivation, reminding you that you're not alone in this voyage.

Visualization is another powerful tool. Envisioning yourself achieving your health goals can be a potent motivator. Imagine the feeling of reaching a desired weight, the sense of pride in managing your blood sugar levels effectively, or the joy of indulging in your favorite activities with renewed vigor. These mental images can serve as beacons of hope and determination, guiding you through rough waters.

Finally, intertwine your diabetes management plan with activities you love. If you enjoy nature, consider outdoor exercises. If cooking is your passion, explore diabetic-friendly recipes. When your health routine aligns with your interests, it doesn't feel like a chore but a part of your lifestyle you embrace with open arms.

In summary, staying motivated in the management of Type 2 Diabetes is about setting personal goals, celebrating small victories, seeking support, visualizing success, and integrating your interests into your health regimen. With these strategies, the journey becomes not just about managing a condition but about living life to its fullest, every step of the way.

Resources for Continued Learning

- **Websites and Online Portals**
  - American Diabetes Association
  - Diabetes UK
  - Centers for Disease Control and Prevention - Diabetes
  - WebMD Diabetes Center
- **Mobile Applications**
  - MySugr: Diabetes Tracker Log
  - Glucose Buddy Diabetes Tracker
  - Carb Manager: Keto Diet App
  - Fooducate - Nutrition Tracker
- **Books and Publications**
  - "The Diabetes Code" by Dr. Jason Fung
  - "Diabetic Living Diabetes Meals by the Plate"
  - "The Complete Diabetes Cookbook" by America's Test Kitchen
  - "The End of Diabetes" by Dr. Joel Fuhrman
- **Support Groups and Forums**
  - Diabetes Daily Forum
  - tudiabetes.org
  - Diabetes.co.uk Forum
  - Children with Diabetes Forums
- **Workshops and Seminars**
  - Diabetes Self-Management Education and Support (DSMES) Services
  - ADA's Diabetes EXPOs
  - Local hospital and clinic-hosted workshops
  - Online webinars by diabetes educators
- **Reputable Health Organizations**
  - National Institute of Diabetes and Digestive and Kidney Diseases (NIDDK)
  - World Health Organization (WHO) - Diabetes
  - International Diabetes Federation (IDF)
  - National Diabetes Education Program (NDEP)

Measurement Conversion Table

Volume Measurements

US Measurement	Metric Measurement
1 teaspoon (tsp)	5 milliliters (ml)
1 tablespoon (tbsp)	15 milliliters (ml)
1 fluid ounce (fl oz)	30 milliliters (ml)
1 cup (C.)	240 milliliters (ml)
1 pint (2 Cs)	470 milliliters (ml)
1 quart (4 Cs)	0.95 liters (L)
1 gallon (16 Cs)	3.8 liters (L)

Weight Measurements

US Measurement	Metric Measurement
1 ounce (oz)	28 grams (g)
1 pound (lb)	450 grams (g)
1 pound (lb)	0.45 kilograms (kg)

Length Measurements

US Measurement	Metric Measurement
1 inch (in)	2.54 centimeters (cm)
1 foot (ft)	30.48 centimeters (cm)
1 foot (ft)	0.3048 meters (m)
1 yard (yd)	0.9144 meters (m)

Temperature Conversions

Fahrenheit (°F)	Celsius (°C)
32°F	0°C
212°F	100°C
Formula: (°F - 32) x 0.5556 = °C	Formula: (°C x 1.8) + 32 = °F

Oven Temperature Conversions

US Oven Term	Fahrenheit (°F)	Celsius (°C)
Very Slow	250°F	120°C
Slow	300-325°F	150-165°C
Moderate	350-375°F	175-190°C
Moderately Hot	400°F	200°C
Hot	425-450°F	220-230°C
Very Hot	475-500°F	245-260°C